Praise for *Miracles We Have Seen*

"As a witness to one of the miracles recounted in this uplifting book, I welcome Dr. Rotbart's extraordinary collection of compelling testimonies from leading physicians. Take a look, and have your faith in God—and in his agents of healing, doctors—renewed!"

—Timothy Michael Cardinal Dolan, Archbishop of New York

"We read so many accounts of freak accidents and rare diseases bringing misery into the lives of people who deserve better. That is why it was so refreshing, so soul-restoring to read these accounts of near tragedies that were prevented by human efforts, good will, and caring."

—Rabbi Harold Kushner, author of *When Bad Things Happen to Good People*
and *Nine Essential Things I've Learned About Life*

"In an age of technology and indifference, these remarkable essays inspire wonder, awe, and a sense of pride of being human. They demonstrate that the miracle of miracles is that they do happen when health professionals combine their medical skills with unrelenting devotion to the art of healing."

—Bernard Lown, MD, Nobel Peace Prize recipient on behalf of the International
Physicians for the Prevention of Nuclear War; Emeritus Professor of Medicine,
Harvard School of Public Health; Emeritus Senior Medical Attending,
Brigham and Women's Hospital; Founder of Physicians for Social Responsibility

"The remarkable stories from *Miracles We Have Seen* will stay with you long after you have put the book down. You will be moved to tears and share in the joy, and sometimes sorrow, experienced by the dedicated doctors who deal with life-and-death issues every day. Modern medicine goes far beyond technology; it is the human factor and the personal relationships that make all the difference. The resilience of the patients, the determination of the doctors and their medical teams, and the serendipitous timing of events that can unexpectedly change an outcome will leave you with a sense of awe and optimism."

—Jack Canfield, co-creator of the *Chicken Soup for the Soul* series,
and creator of *The Success Principles* series

"If you need a dose of beauty, hope and encouragement, you'll find it in this collection of essays from doctors on medical miracles—things they've seen while practicing for which they have no explanation, or only an extraordinary one. It's a happy tears book (and all author proceeds go to charity)."

—KJ Dell'Antonia, *New York Times* columnist and contributing editor; author, "How It's Done" blog

"A collection of essays from top medical professionals in various disciplines that showcase patient outcomes that have defied all expectations and, in many cases, scientific explanations. The essays are written with a blend of technical detail, which fully explains the miraculous events, and a conversational appeal to the unknown, which will engage readers who feel there is more to life than the empirically verifiable . . . Incredibly broad, both in the specialties represented and in the types of miraculous events described, this collection captures the hope that captivated those who experienced the events firsthand . . . the experiences and perspectives this book contains are sure to provide inspiration."

—*Publishers Weekly*

"A beautifully written collection from physicians witnessing the mystery and power of the human body and spirit in the most extreme circumstances. This is a unique contribution that will inspire and edify."

—Jerome Groopman, MD, Recanati Professor, Harvard Medical School,
New Yorker staff writer, and co-author with Dr. Pamela Hartzband of the
New York Times bestseller *Your Medical Mind: How to Decide What Is Right for You*

"Miracles are all around we just need to pause and be still, and recognize them. This book is a testament to the medical miracles that happen every day when skill, science, and spirituality meet."

—Rev. Mpho A. Tutu van Furth, Executive Director, Desmond & Leah Tutu
Legacy Foundation and co-author, with Archbishop Desmond Tutu, of *Made for Goodness*

"*Miracles We Have Seen* opens a window into the complex world of the art and the science of medicine for all to see the compassionate miracles dispensed there. Take a good look . . . you will be inspired!"

—Richard Carmona, MD, MPH, FACS, 17th Surgeon General of the United States

"This is one of the best books I have ever read. The stories in this book will make you want to cry, cheer, embrace, pause and reflect on the miracles that occur each and every day. What a wonderful gift to all of us, captured in this timeless treasure."

—Michelle B. Riba, MD, MS, past President, American Psychiatric
Association; Professor, Department of Psychiatry, University of Michigan;
Director, Psych-Oncology Program, University of Michigan Comprehensive Cancer Center

"These stories by doctors who are true healers have moved me to tears and opened my heart. Each, like the great doctor-writer Chekhov, brings to medicine a sense of compassion, deep vulnerability, love and hope for those who suffer, and the ability to acknowledge that human life is a precious gift."

—Ruth Behar, author of *Traveling Heavy: A Memoir in between Journeys* and the
Victor Haim Perera Collegiate Professor of Anthropology, University of Michigan

"Deeply moving and eloquently written, this remarkable collection reminds us how the art and science of medicine intersect with good luck, coincidence, and the unfathomable. For physicians, these essays call to mind our own stories that inspired us toward the healing of our patients."

—Jeremy A. Lazarus, MD, past President, American Medical Association

"For patients, their families, and all the rest of us, *Miracles We Have Seen* is a welcome reminder that even the most dire diagnoses can have happy endings, thanks to the inspiring dedication of doctors."

—Diane Debrovner, Deputy Editor, *Parents* Magazine

"These stories are remarkable—surprising, inspiring, and full of joy and awe. The voices of these doctors remind us—as they remind themselves—of how much we have to learn from the people we care for, and of the importance of acknowledging the elements of good luck, science, care, coincidence, and wonder."

—Perri Klass, MD, Professor of Journalism and Pediatrics, Director, Arthur L. Carter Journalism Institute, New York University

"Doctors tell the human side of medicine in these stories—revealing the heart and soul that go into truly 'caring' care."

—Jimmie C. Holland, MD, Wayne E. Chapman Chair in Psychiatric Oncology, Memorial Sloan-Kettering Cancer Center, author of *The Human Side of Cancer: Living with Hope, Coping with Uncertainty*

"The art of medicine involves empathy and communicating with families in a very personal way. The science of medicine requires understanding how evidence from well-designed research transforms patient care. The vignettes in this book are at the interface between the art and science. They touch our human spirit in such a profound and inspirational way. This remarkable book shows the humility with which medicine should be practiced and how fortunate physicians are to have such meaningful experiences."

—Stephen Berman, MD, past President, American Academy of Pediatrics; Director, Center for Global Health, Colorado School of Public Health; Professor, University of Colorado School of Medicine and School of Public Health

"These fascinating and inspiring stories reinforce the remarkable things that medical care can do, as well as what is out of our control as clinicians. They remind us of the limits of our knowledge, just as they keep us in awe of the unpredictability of human illness and health."

—Steven E. Weinberger, MD, Executive Vice President and CEO, American College of Physicians

"These powerful and true stories by physicians offer hope from where faith intersects with science and real healing begins."

—Jeffrey J. Cain, MD, past President, American Academy of Family Physicians

"The drive to understand cause and effect is central to human nature. But so, too, is awe in the face of mystery, fate, and the ineffable. The kaleidoscopic collection of stories that fills this volume evokes such awe. Miracles of life and death viewed through the lens of medical science make our lives richer for all that cannot be explained, for the wonder of that which is just beyond our grasp."

—Larry Kramer, President, The William and Flora Hewlett Foundation, former Dean, Stanford Law School

"A remarkable volume of essays detailing prolonged effort and novel therapies leading to miraculous outcomes. Empathic care, co-produced by extraordinary teams of medical professionals, their patients and families. Every page speaks 'gratitude.' These stories will contribute powerfully to cures, and equally to cures of burn-out and despair."

—Richard I. Levin, MD, President and CEO, The Arnold P. Gold Foundation; Emeritus Professor of Medicine, New York and McGill Universities

"The glory of medicine is the hope and inspiration that it provides to all, to save lives, to preserve spirits, to truly help humanity. This book captures the individual spirits of the families and the physicians. We devote ourselves to the families impacted by diseases and tragedy, and feel everlasting gratitude to the physicians providing care at the most difficult of times. This motivating book lifts all of our spirits. It gives examples of adversity, and then instills faith and a sense of triumph. The human spirit truly prevails."

—Jeanne A. Conry, MD, PhD, past President, The American Congress of Obstetricians and Gynecologists; Assistant Physician-in-Chief, The Permanente Medical Group

"At a time when the labor of the ideal physician is described as routinized and industrialized—standard work leading to standard outcomes—these stories inspire. These wise physicians remind us that we are at our best when we are open to the surprises, the graces, and even the miracles that occur when we are present for the ill."

—Abraham M. Nussbaum, MD, MTS, Chief Education Officer, Denver Health; Associate Director of Medical Education, Department of Psychiatry, University of Colorado; and author of *The Finest Traditions of My Calling: One Physician's Search for the Renewal of Medicine*

"To practice medicine means that we physicians keep trying to get better. The leading edge for new treatment approaches sometimes emerges from collections of inspiring case reports like these. Let us integrate the mysterious into medical scientific thinking by acknowledging that we are all part of a greater consciousness and that serendipity and synchronicity can highlight the way."

—Bernard Beitman, MD, author of *Connecting with Coincidence*

MIRACLES WE HAVE SEEN

America's Leading Physicians
Share Stories They Can't Forget

HARLEY A. ROTBART, MD

Health Communications, Inc.
Deerfield Beach, Florida

www.hcibooks.com

Other Books by Dr. Rotbart

940 Saturdays

No Regrets Parenting

Germ Proof Your Kids

The On Deck Circle of Life

Human Enterovirus Infections

Bitter Creek written by Bernie Leadon
© Likely Story Music
Used By Permission. All Rights Reserved.

**Library of Congress Cataloging-in-Publication Data
is available through the Library of Congress**

© 2016 Harley Rotbart, MD

ISBN-13: 978-07573-1937-2 (Paperback)
ISBN-10: 07573-1937-8 (Paperback)
ISBN-13: 978-07573-1938-9 (ePub)
ISBN-10: 07573-1938-6 (ePub)

Publisher: Health Communications, Inc.
        3201 S.W. 15th Street
        Deerfield Beach, FL 33442–8190

Cover and interior design by Lawna Patterson Oldfield
Cover and author photos by Sara Rotbart

*To my wife, Sara, and to
our kids, Matt and Nurit, Emily, and Sam,
each a miracle in his or her own way.*

*To our grandson Gideon for the joy and wonder
he brings to all of us each day.*

*To Samantha and Eitan
for their friendship and love.*

*And in memory of Uncle Donald and Lizzy,
who started this book with me but
couldn't help finish it.*

As soon as man does not take his existence for granted, but beholds it as something unfathomably mysterious, thought begins.

—*Dr. Albert Schweitzer*
(1875–1965)

CONTENTS

7 CHAPTER 1. SPECTACULAR SERENDIPITY

The elevator door opened and out fell a priest in full cardiac arrest. The location of that elevator, and the identity of the person waiting for it on the other side of the doors, could not have been more fortuitous.

Volunteering as he did for many years as a "pretend" patient helping medical students learn to perform a physical exam, the topic of this session became too real for this man. This is the story of a student, a teacher, a surgeon, and a volunteer who that day became a real patient.

In the devastation that was Haiti following the 2010 earthquake, a tiny clinic in an impoverished village received a donated EKG machine that was broken on arrival. This is the story of three teens and the miracles they made possible with that machine.

A forty-year-old infertility patient gave up on her prayers of conceiving after many years and many tries at in vitro fertilization. Unbeknownst to her or her doctors, though, she did conceive. Then the unthinkable happened.

saying their good-byes, the woman's family left her bedside in tears, holding hands and deep in prayer.

ACKNOWLEDGMENTS

First and foremost, I am grateful to my patients and to the patients of the other physician-essayists in this volume. It is through our patients' perseverance and courage, and the trust they and their families have placed in us, that we were privileged to witness the remarkable events described in this book.

Next, my profound gratitude to my esteemed colleagues who graciously shared their most moving and meaningful experiences with me and allowed me to share them with you. The commitment these physicians felt when caring for their most challenging patients, many of whom had dire prognoses, was rewarded with the wonderment those same physicians felt when the outcomes didn't match the predictions. The ability of my colleagues to express both their commitment and their wonderment is what has made this book the achievement that it is. I am also grateful to them for entrusting me to fine-tune their essays and for working so closely with me, often through multiple drafts and phone calls, to find the right words to describe their experiences and express their feelings so sensitively and thoughtfully.

On the practical side, books don't become books without special people behind the scenes. I am very grateful to my literary agent and friend, Lisa Leshne (The Leshne Agency), who has believed in me since the beginning of our work together years ago. My editor at HCI Books, Christine Belleris, and I found a close connection from the very beginning stages of this book, and that connection has only deepened with time as we have worked together to compile this finished product. Thanks also to the fine team at HCI for bringing this book to fruition, including Kim Weiss, Larissa Henoch, Lawna Patterson Oldfield, and Mary Ellen Hettinger. I'm grateful to the following people for their energy and their generosity of spirit in helping with everything from individual essays to the entire project: Deirdre Smerillo, Jamie Kalikow, Jenny Watson Willits, Katie Goodwin, Kristin Connor, Ludmila Kuhilin, Josh Barney, Linda Kamateh, Lindee Donahue, Evan Dechtman, Marlize Scheider, Michael Ferlazzo, Michael Rofe, David Meketon, Jerry Topczewski, Kim Griffith, Winifred King, Denise Nazzaro, Dr. David Elpern, Dr. William Woods, Dr. Mark Ratain, Dr. Tom Howard, Dr. Spencer Kubo, and Dr. Stephen Daniels.

Finally, my deepest thanks to my mom, my late dad, my wife's parents, and the rest of my family and friends who have been miraculous in the love and support they have shown me.

H. A. R.

CONTRIBUTORS

Kenneth G. Adams, MD, Senior Cardiologist and Medical Director, Pentucket Medical Associates, Haverhill, Massachusetts

David Addiss, MD, MPH, Director, Children Without Worms, Task Force for Global Health; Adjunct Professor, Department of Global Health, Rollins School of Public Health, Emory University, Atlanta, Georgia; Adjunct Professor, Eck Institute for Global Health, University of Notre Dame, South Bend, Indiana

Dale S. Adler, MD, Professor of Medicine, Harvard Medical School; Executive Vice Chair, Department of Medicine, Cardiovascular Division, Brigham and Women's Hospital

Philip S. Barie, MD, MBA, Master CCM, Professor of Surgery, Professor of Public Health in Medicine, Weill Cornell Medicine, New York-Presbyterian Hospital/Weill Cornell Medical Center, New York, NY

Trevor J. Bayliss, MD, Hematologist-Oncologist, Berkshire Medical Center

Meredith Belber, MD, Internal Medicine, Corporate Health and Immediate Care Physician, Northwestern Medical Group

Joann N. Bodurtha, MD, MPH, Professor of Pediatrics and Oncology, McKusick-Nathans Institute of Genetic Medicine of the Johns Hopkins University School of Medicine

Denise Bratcher, DO, Professor of Pediatrics, Director, Pediatric Residency Program; University of Missouri–Kansas City School of Medicine and Children's Mercy Hospital

Robert J. Buys, MD, Ophthalmologist, Oregon Health Sciences University, Kaiser Permanente

Mark F. Cotton, MMed (Paed), PhD, Professor, Stellenbosch University and Tygerberg Children's Hospital, Children's Infectious Diseases Clinical Research Unit, Department of Paediatrics and Child Health, Cape Town, South Africa

Claudette Dalton, MD, Assistant Dean Emeritus, University of Virginia School of Medicine; former Chair, American Medical Association Council on Medical Education

Kay Daniels, MD, Clinical Professor of Obstetrics and Gynecology, Stanford University School of Medicine

Clara Escuder, MD, Pediatrician and Integrative Medicine Specialist, York, Pennsylvania

Kathleen Farrell, MD, Assistant Professor of Pediatrics, University of Missouri–Kansas City School of Medicine and Children's Mercy Hospital

Michael Fleischer, MD, Obstetrician-Gynecologist; Chairman, Boca Raton Regional Hospital

Sandra L. Friedman, MD, MPH, Professor of Pediatrics, Section Head, Neurodevelopmental and Behavioral Pediatrics, University of Colorado School of Medicine and Children's Hospital Colorado

Jeremy Garrett, MD, Professor of Pediatrics, Division of Critical Care Medicine; St. Louis University School of Medicine at SSM Health–Cardinal Glennon Children's Hospital

Bradley A. George, MD, Assistant Professor of Pediatrics, Emory University School of Medicine; Division of Pediatric Hematology/Oncology

Philip L. Glick, MD, MBA, Professor of Surgery, Pediatrics, and Management of the Jacobs School of Medicine and Biomedical Sciences and School of Management, State University of New York at Buffalo; Vice Chairman for Finance, Department of Surgery

Mary P. Glode, MD, Professor and Vice Chair Emerita of Pediatrics, University of Colorado School of Medicine and Children's Hospital Colorado; former Section Head, Infectious Diseases

Edward J. Goldson, MD, Professor of Pediatrics, University of Colorado School of Medicine and Children's Hospital Colorado

Lia Gore, MD, Professor of Pediatrics, Medical Oncology and Hematology, University of Colorado School of Medicine; Chief, Pediatric Hematology/ Oncology/Bone Marrow Transplant; The Robert J. and Kathleen A. Clark and Ergen Family Endowed Chairs, Children's Hospital Colorado

Debra Gussman, MD, Obstetrics and Gynecology, Meridian Health, Jersey Shore University Medical Center

M. Kathleen Gutierrez, MD, Associate Professor of Pediatrics Emerita, Lucile Packard Children's Hospital/Stanford University School of Medicine

Harvey Guttmann, MD, Chief of Gastroenterology, Abington Memorial Hospital; President of Gastrointestinal Associates, Inc.

Simon J. Hambidge, MD, PhD, Professor of Pediatrics, University of Colorado School of Medicine; Professor of Epidemiology, University of Colorado School of Public Health; Chief Ambulatory Care Officer, Denver Health

Fred M. Henretig, MD, Professor Emeritus of Pediatrics, Perelman School of Medicine, University of Pennsylvania; Attending Physician and Senior Toxicologist, Division of Emergency Medicine and The Poison Control Center, Children's Hospital of Philadelphia

Joanne M. Hilden, MD, Professor and Associate Section Head, Division of Pediatric Hematology/Oncology/BMT, University of Colorado School of Medicine; Medical Director, Center for Cancer and Blood Disorders, Children's Hospital Colorado

Benjamin Honigman, MD, Professor and Founding Chair of Emergency Medicine; Associate Dean, Clinical Outreach, University of Colorado School of Medicine

Jeffrey S. Hyams, MD, Professor of Pediatrics, University of Connecticut School of Medicine; Head, Division of Digestive Diseases, Hepatology, and Nutrition, Connecticut Children's Medical Center

Daniel Hyman, MD, MMM, Associate Professor, University of Colorado School of Medicine; Chief Quality and Patient Safety Officer, Children's Hospital Colorado

Mary Anne Jackson, MD, Professor and Associate Chair of Community and Regional Pediatric Collaboration, University of Missouri–Kansas City School of Medicine and Children's Mercy Hospital & Clinics; Director, Division of Infectious Diseases

Richard Jacobs, MD, Professor and Chairman, Department of Pediatrics; University of Arkansas for Medical Sciences, Arkansas Children's Hospital, and Arkansas Children's Hospital Research Institute

Richard Johnston Jr., MD, Professor of Pediatrics and Associate Dean for Research Development, University of Colorado School of Medicine; former Chairman of Pediatrics, Children's Hospital of Philadelphia; former Medical Director, March of Dimes

Ryan Jones, MD, Resident Physician, Radiation Oncology, University of Texas Southwestern

Michael S. Kappy, MD, Professor of Pediatrics, University of Colorado School of Medicine and Children's Hospital Colorado

Celia Kaye, MD, PhD, Professor Emerita of Pediatrics and former Senior Associate Dean for Education, University of Colorado School of Medicine; Professor Emerita of Pediatrics and former Chair of Pediatrics, University of Texas Health Science Center at San Antonio

David Keller, MD, Professor of Pediatrics and Vice Chair of Clinical Affairs and Clinical Transformation, University of Colorado School of Medicine and Children's Hospital Colorado

David Kimberlin, MD, Professor and Vice Chair for Clinical and Translational Research, Co-Director, Division of Infectious Diseases, University of Alabama at Birmingham; Director, Collaborative Antiviral Study Group, National Institutes of Health

Richard D. Krugman, MD, Professor of Pediatrics, former Vice Chancellor and Dean, University of Colorado School of Medicine

Richard L. Lambert, MD, Assistant Professor of Pediatrics, Temple University School of Medicine; Director, Pediatric Sedation Service, Associate Director, Pediatric Critical Care Medicine, Janet Weis Children's Hospital at Geisinger Health System

Barbara Laughton, MBChB, DCH, MSc, Developmental Pediatrician, Stellenbosch University and Tygerberg Children's Hospital, Children's Infectious Diseases Clinical Research Unit, Department of Paediatrics and Child Health, Cape Town, South Africa

Michael D. Lockshin, MD, Professor of Medicine and Obstetrics-Gynecology, Weill Cornell Medicine; Director, Barbara Volcker Center, Hospital for Special Surgery; formerly Acting Director, National Institute of Arthritis and Musculoskeletal and Skin Diseases, National Institutes of Health

Stephen Ludwig, MD, Professor of Pediatrics and Emergency Medicine, University of Pennsylvania Perelman School of Medicine; Medical Director, International Medical Education, The Children's Hospital of Philadelphia

Frank Maffei, MD, Vice Chairman, Department of Pediatrics, Medical Director, Pediatric Intensive Care Unit, Associate Professor of Pediatrics; Janet Weis Children's Hospital at Geisinger Health System; Temple University School of Medicine

Matthew Metz, MD, Chief, Bariatric Surgery, Parker Adventist Hospital

John W. Ogle, MD, Professor and Vice Chair Emeritus of Pediatrics, University of Colorado School of Medicine; former Director of Pediatrics, Denver Health

Matthew Old, MD, Assistant Professor, Department of Otolaryngology (Head and Neck Surgery), Ohio State University, James Cancer Hospital and Solove Research Institute

David M. Polaner, MD, Professor of Anesthesiology and Pediatrics, Director of Pediatric Transplant Anesthesia, University of Colorado School of Medicine and Children's Hospital Colorado

Mortimer Poncz, MD, Jane Fishman Grinberg Endowed Chair in Stem Cell Research; Professor of Pediatrics and Division Chief, Pediatric Hematology, Perelman School of Medicine, University of Pennsylvania and Children's Hospital of Philadelphia

Valerie Pruitt, MD, Medical Director Trauma and Surgical Intensive Care, Sacred Heart Hospital, Pensacola, Florida

Eugenia Raichlin, MD, Associate Professor of Medicine, University of Nebraska Medical Center

Bruce Reidenberg, MD, Medical Specialist 2 [Senior Physician]; New York State Office for People with Developmental Disabilities

Frank O. Richards Jr., MD, Director, River Blindness Elimination Program, The Carter Center, Emory University School of Medicine

Bruce L. Ring, MD, Internist, Steward Medical Group, Boston, Massachusetts

Mary Catherine Finn Ring, RN, MSN, PNP-C, Pediatric Nurse Practitioner, Village Pediatrics, Brockton, Massachusetts

Richard Roberts, MD, Neurosurgeon, Cook Children's Hospital, Ft. Worth, Texas

Harley A. Rotbart, MD, Professor and Vice Chair Emeritus of Pediatrics, University of Colorado School of Medicine and Children's Hospital Colorado

Ann Schongalla, MD, Assistant Attending Psychiatrist, New York–Presbyterian Hospital; Weill Cornell Medicine

Andrew Sirotnak, MD, Professor and Vice Chair of Pediatrics, University of Colorado School of Medicine and Children's Hospital Colorado

Paul A. Skudder, MD, Clinical Adjunct Assistant Professor of Surgery, Uniformed Services University of the Health Sciences; Cape Cod Healthcare, Falmouth Hospital

David Slamowitz, MD, Medical Director, The SleepWell Center, Denver, Colorado

Henry Sondheimer, MD, Professor and Associate Dean Emeritus, University of Colorado School of Medicine and Children's Hospital Colorado; former Senior Director for Medical Education Projects, Association of American Medical Colleges

David Spiegel, MD, Willson Professor and Associate Chair of Psychiatry and Behavioral Sciences, Stanford University School of Medicine; Director of the Center on Stress and Health, and Medical Director of the Center for Integrative Medicine at Stanford

Alan R. Spitzer, MD, Senior Vice President for Research, Education, and Quality, MEDNAX Services/Pediatrix Medical Group/American Anesthesiology, Sunrise, Florida

Christopher Stille, MD, MPH, Professor and Section Head of General Academic Pediatrics, University of Colorado School of Medicine and Children's Hospital Colorado

Carol L. Storey-Johnson, MD, Associate Professor of Clinical Medicine and Senior Advisor, Medical Education; former Senior Associate Dean (Education); Weill Cornell Medicine

Anthony Suchman, MD, MA, Clinical Professor of Medicine, University of Rochester School of Medicine and Dentistry; Founder and Senior Consultant, Relationship Centered Health Care

Bauer Sumpio, MD, PhD, Professor of Surgery (Vascular) and Diagnostic Radiology; Emeritus Chief, Vascular Surgery; Associate Director, Graduate Medical Education; Yale School of Medicine

James K. Todd, MD, Professor and Vice Chair of Pediatrics, Professor of Microbiology and Epidemiology, University of Colorado School of Medicine and Children's Hospital Colorado; Section Head, Epidemiology

Gilbert R. Upchurch Jr., MD, Professor of Surgery and Chief, Division of Vascular and Endovascular Surgery, University of Virginia School of Medicine

Adrienne Weiss-Harrison, MD, Director of Health Services, City School District of New Rochelle, NY; American Academy of Pediatrics Council on School Health Executive Committee; American Lung Association of the Northeast Board of Directors

Richard Westcott, MA, BM, BCh, DRCOG, DCH, Physician and Teacher in General Practice, South Molton Devon, United Kingdom

Rodney E. Willoughby, MD, Professor of Pediatrics, Medical College of Wisconsin and Children's Hospital of Wisconsin

Amanda Yeaton-Massey, MD, Resident in Obstetrics, Stanford University School of Medicine

INTRODUCTION

Physicians hold a privileged place in their patients' lives, sharing times of great joy and times of great sorrow. To earn this special role, we prepare for many years. In college, we study the basic sciences: biology, chemistry, physics, and others. We move on to medical school for the clinically relevant sciences, including anatomy, biochemistry, pathology, physiology, microbiology, and more. Outside the lecture halls and labs, we shadow senior physicians on clinical rotations through all the medical specialties: internal medicine, surgery, pediatrics, obstetrics-gynecology, psychiatry, family medicine, neurology. But we're still not finished. After choosing a field for our careers, we undertake a grueling apprenticeship called internship and residency that lasts several years, and we often follow that with further subspecialty training in a fellowship.

After all those years learning and training, digesting thousands of textbook pages and medical journal articles, listening to hundreds of lectures, and encountering countless real patients with real diseases and injuries, it would be reasonable to assume doctors understand just about everything there is to understand about the workings of the human body. Yet, in the daily practice of medicine, physicians are often surprised. Two patients with the same diagnosis each have nuances that distinguish them. Illnesses that are usually predictable take unexpected twists and turns. Treatments have unanticipated consequences. Patients and their families amaze us with seemingly impossible inner fortitude and resilience in the face of tragedy and grief. Physicians are accustomed to expect the unexpected, and we are usually well-prepared to respond.

1

But occasionally in the course of caring for our patients, we encounter events that truly stun us: unforgettable occurrences that defy all of our predictions and expectations, far exceeding the wide berth we are trained to allow for surprise. These are events for which there is no clear medical or psychological explanation, or if there is, the explanation itself is extraordinary. When these occur, we are rarely alone in our awe; medicine is a collaborative endeavor, so during these truly confounding and mysterious episodes, we seek advice and consultation from colleagues, specialists, and mentors. And when they, too, are at a loss to explain what we are seeing, the experience often deeply impacts everyone involved.

This book tells the stories of medical "miracles" in the words of leading doctors who witnessed them, physicians at the top of their fields. Contributors to this book include pediatricians, internists, surgeons, family medicine specialists, emergency medicine physicians, obstetricians, psychiatrists, and subspecialists in a wide variety of fields. They include leaders in the bedside care of individual patients, as well as in global health care where entire populations are affected. Among our essayists are dozens of preeminent educators, including deans and department heads, on the faculties of the top university medical schools in the country. All of our essayists also care for patients, spanning the broad clinical spectrum from community practitioners to highly specialized experts at major medical centers. The common thread among us is that we have borne witness to unexplainable, unforgettable, and profoundly unexpected events—medical miracles—in our patients.

These are not miracles resulting solely from heroic or high-tech medical interventions, situations for which we have a good explanation for the outcome—thoughtful, caring, and talented medical personnel applying state-of-the-art technology to save lives. Rather, the stories in this book are of patients whose outcomes amazed their doctors and nurses, perhaps *despite* their heroic efforts, because of the seeming impossibility of the events that took place. The stories recount spectacular serendipities, impossible cures, breathtaking resuscitations, extraordinary awakenings, and recovery from unimaginable disasters. Still other essays tell of physicians' experiences in which the miracle was more emotional than physical, yet also left a lasting imprint. Doctors sharing in gut-wrenching decisions made by patients and families, and then in the resulting joy—or heartbreak. Discovering a silver lining of forgiveness or resilience, a child's wisdom or a family's generosity of spirit, evoked salvation and triumph in the face of sadness and tragedy. Over the course of a career, these emotionally stunning events occur more frequently than, for example, a patient "coming back to life" or recovering from a terminal disease after all hope had been lost, yet they are no less inspirational, no less miraculous to those witnessing them. As my colleague and friend Dr. Kevin Kalikow commented, it's those essays that truly illustrate the difference between "curing" and "healing."

The first medical miracle I witnessed was as a pediatrics resident-in-training. Two young brothers, ages three and seven, were brought into the emergency room and then the intensive care unit after near-drowning episodes. The recovery of one of the brothers was so unlikely, so astounding, that I was forever imprinted by the experience. This was not the last miracle I would see in my thirty-plus years as a pediatrics specialist. Many of my colleagues would agree that, despite being at the forefront of medicine and science, what we *don't* understand often exceeds what we *do* understand. And even when we think we understand, we are frequently proven wrong.

The word "miracle" is often used in religious contexts, and while faith and prayer certainly play an important role in many of our patients' lives, as well as in some of the vignettes in this compilation, this is not a book about religion. I will leave it to the reader to determine what, if any, role those factors play in the outcome of these stories. Rather, this is a book about optimism and inspiration, and the realization that what we don't know or don't understand isn't necessarily cause for fear, and can even be reason for hope.

The experience of inviting physicians to contribute essays to this collection has, in and of itself, been enlightening for me. There have been three general categories of responses, all very thoughtful in their own way. Some colleagues knew right away that they hadn't had "miraculous experiences," and politely thanked me for asking. A second group said, "Nothing comes to mind right away, but I'll keep thinking on it and try to come up with something." With only a few exceptions, those physicians didn't have a belated epiphany despite pondering it. The third group of responses was most exciting for me. These colleagues immediately replied with, "Oh my goodness! I have an amazing story I've been waiting for the chance to tell." Not all of us are fortunate enough to encounter unexplained, unexpected, deeply moving and mysterious moments in medicine. But when a medical miracle—physical, emotional, or both—does occur in a physician's career, it's unforgettable, in the forefront of our minds, and ripe for telling. In the telling of the inspirational stories that fill this book, we learn as much about the physicians as about their patients. My editor at HCI Books, Christine Belleris, said it beautifully: Emerging through all of the moving personal testimonials from physicians in this collection is a compelling glimpse into the lives and souls of doctors—their compassion, humanity, and determined devotion to their patients and their patients' families.

The other striking observation for me regarding the essays is how many of the events occurred decades earlier—often in the early stages of a physician's training or practice. This is another testament to the powerful impact these experiences have on those witnessing them—unforgettable, still affecting physicians' personal and professional lives. In these decades-old cases, the essayist-physician often recalls the concomitant astonished reactions of his or her senior and supervising physicians, expressed on rounds and in case conferences. It was the astonishment of the senior physicians, highly trained specialists and experienced mentors, as much as the amazement felt by the young physicians, that kept those memories alive all these years. In many cases, physicians describing events occurring years ago noted that those early memories served to give them hope as they encountered new, seemingly hopeless cases in subsequent years. Some contributors wrote that the miracle experience actually directed them in their choice of specialty and has influenced much of their professional decision-making throughout their careers. Others draw on those miraculous moments at times when they themselves feel helpless in the face of adversity and tragedy. Powerful stuff.

Another unexpected and quite magical outgrowth of this project has been the reconnections that some of the physician-essayists have now made with the patients and patients' families with whom they shared the miracle years earlier. Either in the course of tracking down the individuals for permission to tell their story, or simply reaching out to learn what has become of them, writing these essays has renewed old bonds. These reconnections have been moving and gratifying for everyone involved—including me, when I've been privileged to be included in the conversation.

Finally, three especially noteworthy responses to my invitation to submit an essay deserve special mention:

Several colleagues responded by saying that their memories of patients whose outcomes were unexpectedly *bad* are more vivid and haunting than those with miraculously *good* outcomes. That is only natural—we all relive and replay the horrible stories, asking ourselves, *What went wrong?* and *What more could I have done?* We must accept the inevitability of bad things occasionally happening to our patients over which we have no more control than we do over mystifyingly good outcomes like some of those described in this book. And among other essays herein, particularly those in the "Silver Linings" chapter, a mix of good and bad can occur with potent outcomes. Over the course of our careers, we can only hope that the positive results outweigh the negative, sustaining us in the good works we hope to accomplish.

Two essay contributors asked me to caution readers that patients' dependence on miracles can be detrimental. While retaining hope in seemingly hopeless situations is emotionally and sometimes even physically healing, hope alone will not cure disease. When proven medical treatments are available and beneficial, but declined in favor of waiting for a miracle, the patient will likely be disappointed. The takeaway message from the essays in this book cannot be to rely solely on a bolt of lightning from above. I received no essays for this collection of miraculous outcomes describing patients who refused proven medical therapy. My grandfather used to tell a joke about the saintly but impoverished old man who prayed and prayed and prayed to win the lottery so he could live a better life in his last years. After years of having his prayers unfulfilled, he finally threw up his hands and asked, "Dear Lord, I have been a good servant for many years, doing good for others while sacrificing my own needs. Why haven't you granted my wish to win the lottery?" In a booming voice from heaven, the response came, "My son, you have to buy a ticket!" Hoping for the best outcome possible in a time of medical crisis is natural and uplifting, but you have to buy a ticket—if established and effective therapies are available, don't ignore them while waiting for a miracle.

And in the third notable response to my invitation, two colleagues expressed nearly identical sentiments, quoted here with their permission. Although neither had a singularly "miraculous" patient experience to relate, Nathan Rabinovitch, MD, Professor of Pediatrics at the University of Colorado School of Medicine, said, "Doing what we do as doctors, and seeing all that can go wrong, I've come to appreciate that every healthy day is a miracle." And Allan Gibofsky, Professor of Medicine at Weill Cornell Medicine, answered, "The longer I live, the more convinced I am that every breath, every heartbeat (and yes, even every bowel movement) is itself a miracle. We spend so much of our professional lives as doctors dealing with what is wrong in our patients (and ourselves), that I fear we have become inured to appreciating all that goes right." Amen to both of them.

Thank you for giving audience to the stories we've been waiting to tell about the miracles we've been so fortunate to see.

—Harley A. Rotbart, MD

1

Spectacular Serendipity

When an inconceivable event takes place, sometimes it's hard to know if the event itself is miraculous or if the timing of the event is the true miracle. Did the Red Sea miraculously split or were the ancient Hebrews miraculously at its shore precisely when a naturally occurring phenomenon began?

The essays in this chapter describe extraordinary medical outcomes that could only have occurred exactly when and where they did.

DATE OF EVENT: 1988

Father Karl's Miraculous Timing

Dale S. Adler, MD

I t was a Saturday afternoon at an urban academic medical center. I'm a cardiologist, and was on call for the coronary care unit (CCU, the intensive care unit for heart patients) and the cardiac catheterization laboratory (commonly known as the "cath lab") where we do dye studies to evaluate the blood vessels of the heart. As beautiful a day as it was outside, I knew I was not likely to enjoy much of the blue sky and sunshine. I had just finished an emergent case in the cath lab and I was happy for the nurses and technician there, who were hurriedly putting away equipment and making their computer entries. They might still be able to enjoy the waning hours of sunlight with their families. I let them know that all seemed quiet and they should try to get out of the hospital.

I was waiting for an elevator on the second floor that housed both the cath lab and the CCU, on my way upstairs to see a hospitalized patient. I intended to return to the CCU later to finish rounding on the patients I had admitted there earlier that day.

The elevator doors opened and, to my utter astonishment and great dismay, a body rolled forward over the threshold. Gray hair, overweight, black suit. Entirely unconscious based on the roll. I turned the man over, face up. Others who were also waiting for the elevator helped me. Priest's collar, pulseless, sweaty, clammy—drenched, in fact—cold, pale. We started CPR (cardiopulmonary resuscitation), and someone notified the hospital operator to broadcast a call mobilizing the emergency response team, but we didn't wait for them to arrive. We dragged the lifeless body, while still doing CPR, toward the cath lab. More help arrived, with a gurney and defibrillator machine—the paddles for shocking the heart back to life that you see on all those hospital TV shows. Quick check of his heart rhythm: *fine ventricular fibrillation*, the most ominous heart pattern—his heart was doing virtually nothing. Shocked him with the paddles. No help. Quick lift onto the gurney, and we rolled him into the cath lab.

Fortunately, the cath lab nurses and technician had heard the call for the emergency response team and had not left the hospital. They were at the ready. Like a well-trained orchestra, everyone did their job. We learned that our patient was Father Karl, a popular seventy-year-old priest whose church and followers were about a thirty-minute drive from the hospital. Father Karl had been dutifully visiting his hospitalized parishioners, offering prayers of healing. We knew none of his medical history. We had no idea how long he had been pitched up against the elevator door. We didn't know on which floor he had entered the elevator, nor why it stopped on our cardiac floor. We only knew he was cold and clammy and pulseless when he rolled forward from the elevator. His pupils were fixed and dilated, a very bad sign of impending death and/or brain damage. This was in an era long before we knew about cooling to protect the brain.

With ongoing CPR, we performed a catheterization procedure to find the cause of his cardiac arrest in hopes of reversing it. The procedure involves inserting a catheter (tube) into a large vein that runs directly to the heart. Dye is then injected into the arteries of the heart to find the problem. The large main artery on the front of the heart was occluded by a clot. That was the cause of his heart attack—that main artery is colloquially known as the "widow maker" because when it's blocked, there's big trouble.

While visualizing the catheterization procedure on the video monitor, I was able to reach his blocked artery with the catheter and slide a wire, and then a balloon, across the soft clot. I dilated the balloon to open up the artery, and then deflated it. Blood flow in the vessel was restored. This was at a time before stent devices, which these days are left in the opened arteries to keep them open, but the flow through his artery continued to look strong after the balloon procedure. He was still without a heartbeat. Another shock with the paddles, now to a heart getting adequate blood flow, was followed by return of a more normal heart rhythm, and then a weak but definite pulse. We boosted his blood pressure with another type of device, this one inserted into his aorta (the main artery leaving the heart), and with multiple medications.

I was told that people were in the waiting area, wanting to know about Father Karl's condition. I arrived there, my scrubs soaked with Father Karl's blood and sweat. Some of my own sweat, I presume, as well. I was greeted by a sea of black and white, a roomful of priests and nuns, every seat taken. They had heard about their beloved Father Karl and had come to see him and to pray. They all stood up as I arrived.

I told them that the good news was that Father Karl was alive, at the moment, and in our CCU with a heartbeat and a blood pressure. The blood pressure, of course, was being helped by many medications and the intra-aortic device. The bad news was we had no idea whether Father Karl's brain had survived this dramatic insult. We didn't know if he had been out for sixty seconds or five minutes before the elevator doors opened and we started CPR. The loyal legion said that they would pray for Father Karl and for the physicians. One after another expressed profound gratitude for what we had already done.

A mere four weeks later, after a full recovery, Father Karl addressed his congregation. He expressed gratitude to God and, graciously, to his physicians.

I, too, was very grateful. Grateful that a kind and revered man who had just been bringing good wishes and prayers to patients had the good fortune of having his potentially fatal heart attack in a hospital. More precisely, in a hospital elevator, which opened to the hospital floor where I was standing waiting for that elevator. The same hospital floor where the cardiac cath lab and CCU were located, and where I and others, trained and experienced in just this type of cardiac emergency, were still at work on a weekend day.

Grateful that after literally falling at my feet, as if delivered to me, his heart finally responded to our treatment. Treatment that would have been impossible to receive in such a timely fashion had he collapsed almost anywhere else that day. Grateful that the prayers he said for our patients earlier that day were repaid many times over by the prayers of his community who had gathered in our waiting room that afternoon, and subsequently in his church during the harrowing days that followed.

As the saying goes, timing is everything. I will always be grateful for Father Karl's timing.

DATE OF EVENT: FEBRUARY 2013

An Unlikely Discovery by the Unlikeliest Person

Ryan Jones, MD
Claudette Dalton, MD
Gilbert Upchurch Jr., MD

EDITOR'S NOTE: This remarkable story is separately told by three different caregivers, each from their unique vantage points. The roles of the medical student (Dr. Jones), teacher (Dr. Dalton), and surgeon (Dr. Upchurch) were each essential—without any one of them, the miracle would never have happened.

PART 1. THE STUDENT

In all honesty, I was just trying to pass my exam. Once a week or so for the first two years of medical school, my fellow students and I donned our short white coats and had contact with patients as part of our Clinical Performance Development course. The contact ranged from watching trained physicians interview and examine patients, to doing the same ourselves under the supervision of our physician teachers. On the day that led to this essay, I was at the end of my third year of medical school, feeling fairly relaxed because the "worst" of my difficult rotations were behind me. I was generally comfortable with my skills in obtaining a medical history from a patient and performing a physical examination, and the exercise that day was designed to test those skills in preparation for the national licensing examination I would take in the near future.

The exercise consisted of a series of volunteer pretend "patients," each with a different faux condition, from whom we students were expected to extract the relevant information to lead us to the diagnosis the actors were pretending to have. It was a little like a game—these pretend patients revealed only the information we students elicited by careful questioning. After the questioning, we went through the motions of a physical examination directed at where we thought the problem might be, based on our interview with the patient, and then we summarized our treatment plan to both the patient and a physician proctor for the exam. Once we finished the case, we moved on to the next.

When I walked into Jim's room, I had just finished a previous case where I thought I could have done better. I belatedly realized questions I should have asked and was kicking myself for the mistakes. Nonetheless, I told myself to let it go and focus on the next patient, Jim, a seventy-five-year-old retired engineer. Fortunately, Jim's story was fairly straightforward. He conveyed risk factors in his history for an abdominal aortic aneurysm (an abnormal and potentially dangerous bulge in the aorta, the main artery in the body that courses from the heart through the chest and abdomen), and he reported symptoms that could be explained by a large abdominal mass or aneurysm. When it came time for the physical examination, I knew the abdomen would be my primary focus.

The physical exam of the abdomen is an important part of a physician's education, of course, but I was just focusing on making sure I got all the steps right so the preceptor observing me on closed circuit TV from another room would see I knew what I was doing. In this case, I was going through the motions of looking for an abdominal mass or an abdominal aortic aneurysm. The latter, in particular, can be detected by feeling a pulsating ("beating") mass in the abdomen or by hearing a *bruit*, a sound from turbulent blood flow, with a stethoscope. With Jim, I wasn't expecting to find anything, of course—he was a pretend patient! I vividly recall the *Whoa!* moment when I thought I felt a pulsating mass in Jim's abdomen, right where the aorta should be. I took a step back from the exam table and collected my thoughts. Then, listening to his abdomen, I thought I heard a bruit, adding weight to my diagnosis of an abdominal aortic aneurysm. A real one!

It seemed odd to me that Jim would be volunteering for this case. I thought he must be a "ringer," a patient with an *actual* disease thrown into the test setting to see if the students would detect a real condition—in this case, a very serious one. Rumor had it that sometimes national examiners do that for the licensing tests, but this was just a clinical skills course as part of medical school—highly unlikely to have a patient with a real disease volunteering to play the part for the students in this setting. I was so taken aback by what I felt and heard that I "broke character" for a moment and addressed Jim as a potential real patient rather than a pretend patient. After all, he was report- ing to have symptoms—I needed to be sure that what he was saying wasn't true, because the symptoms he was describing would have raised concern for leakage from the aneurysm or impending rupture, a highly fatal complication.

"Do you know you might have an abdominal aortic aneurysm?"

But Jim stayed in character. "What's an aneurysm?" he asked, even though his job that day was to portray a patient with an abdominal aortic aneurysm and he had been fully prepped in the condition he was "pretending" to have. Later, I learned that all the symptoms Jim had complained about to me were, indeed, pretend, just part of the test. In fact, he never had any symptoms. It turns out that many patients with real abdominal aortic aneurysms don't have symptoms, sometimes until it's too late.

I reported my findings to my preceptor, Dr. Dalton, as part of my responsibility to present the case as a doctor would when discussing a real patient. Dr. Dalton seemed skeptical of my findings of an abdominal aortic aneurysm in a patient who thought he was pretending to have one. I wondered to myself whether it was even safe for a patient with a real aneurysm to have his belly poked and prodded by student after student, but I assumed everyone knew what they were doing, including Jim, and that my concerns were above my pay grade. Keeping in line with the test protocol, I moved on to my next pretend patient of the day. Each of the students saw eight such volunteers in the same day as part of this testing.

When Jim's aneurysm was subsequently confirmed by his physicians and the surgical correction performed, there was quite a media storm[1-4]: "UVA Medical Student Diagnoses Actor with Life-Threatening Condition During Practice Exam." "Med Student Discovers Real Disease in Fake Patient." "U-VA Med Student Saves Man's Life During Training Exam." "Med Student Saves Life of Elderly Man Acting as Pretend Patient." I received congratulatory emails from the president of the university, the dean of the medical school, and the CEO of the hospital.

All the fuss took me by surprise, but I enjoyed getting to share the story with so many people. Really, I was just trying to pass my exam. Most meaningful to me, Jim and his wife were extraordinarily grateful, telling everyone I had saved his life. But, as I told the media, Jim and I were both just fortunate to be in the right place at the right time.

---

1 http://www.cbsnews.com/news/uva-medical-student-diagnoses-actor-with-life-threatening-condition-during-practice-exam/

2 http://abcnews.go.com/Health/med-student-discovers-real-disease-fake-patient/story?id=21475027

3 http://www.washingtonpost.com/blogs/answer-sheet/wp/2014/01/13/u-va-medical-student-saves-mans-life-during-training-exam/

4 http://insider.foxnews.com/2014/01/07/uva-med-student-saves-life-elderly-man-who-was-serving-patient-actor

PART 2. THE TEACHER

I have the privilege of supervising medical students who are early in their training and learning to interview and examine patients for the first time. One of our most effective teaching strategies is with "standardized patients"—local residents who portray a patient scenario for medical students to practice their skills—for little or no pay. These "pretend patients" are prepped on how to give consistent histories and behaviors to all the students who examine them. That is no mean feat when you are allowing dozens of students to question, pummel, and fumble through a history and physical exam.

Jim is a retired executive who has volunteered his time for many years to portray patients with various conditions. Jim's wife also is a standardized patient, and the two of them have a sweet, caring relationship that is a joy to witness. They really enjoy contributing together to medical education in this unique way.

On the day in question, Jim was acting as a patient with a possible leaking *abdominal aortic aneurysm*. (As an aside, his wife was portraying a depressed patient for the students that day.) The aorta is the main artery in the abdomen, and it sometimes develops a defect that causes it to balloon; this balloon is called an aneurysm. As the ballooning aorta grows bigger, it can leak and even rupture—two very serious and potentially lethal complications. The objective for the students examining Jim was to get a history of underlying risk factors for aneurysms, such as high blood pressure, smoking, and disease in other blood vessels, as well as to obtain a history of belly pain. Then the students were expected to do the proper abdominal exam, focusing on findings that might indicate the presence of an aneurysm, such as a mass that was pulsating, a widened aorta, or an abnormal sound of turbulent blood flow called a "bruit."

No one expected there to be real physical findings—after all, the standardized patients portray all sorts of diseases that they don't have and for which they should have no real signs on physical examination. The exercise was to ensure the students asked the right questions in the right way, and went through the motions of the exam correctly. My role was to watch the exam in real time on a closed-circuit TV in another room, and then listen while the student "presented" the patient to me—a test of his or her ability to organize the information and give it back reliably.

Ryan Jones was the last student of the day. I had observed and listened to seven others that day and twenty-four others in the three afternoons that week prior to this session. Hence, Ryan was the thirty-second medical student to examine Jim's belly. Ryan did a nice job on both his history and physical examination and his presentation was also well done. But, when he told me that he had felt a pulsating mass and heard a bruit over the abdominal aorta, I admit to being a little peeved. *He's making that up or imagining it,* I thought. I challenged him, and asked if he was saying that to represent what he would have heard in a real patient. "No," he insisted, "I really felt a mass and heard a bruit!"

Something about Ryan's quiet assurance got me out of the chair from my viewing booth and down the hall to Jim's room. He was already dressed and ready to leave but readily agreed to let me examine his abdomen. And there they were—an unmistakable mass and bruit. *Geez!* I couldn't believe I almost dismissed Ryan's findings as imaginary.

By this time, Jim was looking a bit confused. I told him that Ryan had felt and heard something unusual and that I had confirmed it. My advice was to go to see his primary care doctor sooner rather than later and get an abdominal ultrasound. Jim didn't seem entirely convinced—he felt fine, looked fine, and had taken good care of himself. But he did say I could talk to his wife who was finishing up her "performance" in another examination room. That sweet woman looked her husband in the eyes and started issuing orders—he *would* be going to see his physician. Clearly, this soft-spoken, rosy-cheeked, seventy-plus tiny lady was in charge of the situation. Impressive, especially considering she must have been emotionally and physically exhausted after play-acting as a depressed patient for thirty-two medical students that week alone! I knew she would make her husband do the right thing.

Indeed, Jim's wife marched him straight to his doctor, the aneurysm was confirmed and the surgery was done by Dr. Upchurch. Without Ryan's good exam, his mention of something no one else had heard or felt, and his quiet but confident insistence that it was real, who knows when or if Jim's aneurysm would have been discovered in time?

PART 3: THE SURGEON

I see hundreds of patients a year for surgery on diseased blood vessels, referred from fellow surgeons and other physicians all over Virginia and around the country. But, in my more than twenty years performing vascular surgery, seeing and operating on thousands of patients, I have never received a patient referral like this one, and I doubt I ever will again.

Jim came to me after a medical student named Ryan Jones felt a pulsating mass and heard a "bruit," which is the sound of abnormal turbulent blood flow, in Jim's abdomen. Jones's examination took place as part of our university medical school's "standardized patient" program, wherein volunteers pretend to have a certain condition to help teach our medical students. Jim was supposed to be just an actor, pretending to have an aneurysm so the students could practice their skills. Ryan Jones must have been imagining the findings, right? None of the other students who examined Jim that day felt or heard anything abnormal. Perhaps it was the power of suggestion—Jones knew what he was looking for so he imagined he found it?

No, this was a real aneurysm in a patient pretending to have one. The mass and the bruit sound were confirmed by Dr. Dalton, his proctor for the day, and the patient was referred to me after an ultrasound confirmed the finding. When I evaluated Jim, I observed a thin, fit, and elderly male, the "classic" appearance of patients with abdominal aortic aneurysms. He had no symptoms whatsoever and he was sure this was some kind of mistake. Both he and his wife were nervous about the diagnosis and the treatment that would be required. Indeed, I confirmed the medical student's physical examination findings and the diagnosis of an abdominal aortic aneurysm was confirmed by CAT scan (a special type of X-ray).

Surgery has come a long way for this problem in recent years. In the past, we opened up the abdomen with a large incision and performed a lengthy and risky resection (removal) of the aneurysm and replacement with a tube (graft) made of artificial material. Now, in most patients, we are able to fix the ballooning vessel by snaking what we call an "endograft" into the aorta through a small incision in the patient's groin. The endograft is like the inner tube of a tire—we inflate it within the diseased portion of the aorta and it stabilizes the blood vessel, preventing it from leaking or bursting. I performed this procedure on Jim and he was able to go home the next day without any complications. He was stunned by how this all happened, but he and his wife were very grateful to the medical student, the student's teacher, and me for preventing what could have been a disastrous outcome had the aneurysm not been detected early.

At the time of surgery, Jim had a six centimeter (approximately 2.5 inches) size aneurysm. Aneurysms can grow rapidly. Studies have shown that aneurysms of six centimeters in males have an 8 to 10 percent chance of rupturing each year. The death rate from a ruptured aneurysm is greater than 50 percent. However, if we can fix the aneurysm before it ruptures, as we were able to do with Jim, the death rate is reduced dramatically to only 1 to 5 percent.

Even more remarkably, studies have been done testing skilled physicians' abilities to detect aneurysms in patients who are known to have aneurysms present. Even in the best of hands, physical examination can only detect an aneurysm 50 percent of the time. That's because physical findings of aneurysms and many other conditions can often be subtle, transitory, or absent entirely. The physical examination is as often the "art of medicine" as it is the "science of medicine." Ryan Jones was by no means a skilled examiner—he was still a medical student, early in his training. But he was a medical student with astute observation skills and the confidence to pursue what he believed he discovered, no matter how unlikely it may have been. He may well have saved Jim's life.

It was Jim's good fate to have fallen into this medical student's hands on that particular day. We are blessed to be in this profession.

DATE OF EVENT: 2012

Three Teens and a Miraculous Machine

Mary Catherine Finn Ring, RN, MSN, PNP-C
Bruce Ring, MD

After the devastating 2010 earthquake in Haiti, medical teams from around the world mobilized to provide urgent aid. In the years since, recovery has been glacially slow and medical teams have continued on missions to the battered country. We have been privileged to be among those who have made repeated visits. Our work has been focused in a rural mountain village one hour from Port-au-Prince where a tiny clinic stands, overwhelmed by the needs of the impoverished residents. The village had no running water until 2012. Medical supplies are limited to what we can fly in from the States, which we gather by soliciting donations of medicines and equipment prior to each trip. Typically, each mission is staffed by two medical personnel and several non-medical folks, sometimes including teenagers volunteering through their school.

There is no computer access in this village, and in fact, electricity is only intermittent, as is true almost everywhere in Haiti. As only the most basic lab tests can be performed, such as a simple blood count and a few others, care is delivered mostly based on the practitioners' diagnostic skills.

An electrocardiograph (EKG) machine for testing heart function was desperately needed in that clinic.

TEEN #1—THE ROBOTICS TECHIE

On this particular trip, the team was excited to have procured a donated EKG machine to bring along with them for the clinic. The excitement was short-lived, however, when they arrived with the EKG machine in the clinic only to discover the machine was broken. One of the volunteers on that trip was a student named Daniel who was a member of the robotics club at his high school. Daniel suggested he and his fellow club members might be able to repair the machine, so arrangements were made to bring it back to the States with the team. Sure enough, these tech-savvy high schoolers, who had never before worked with an EKG machine or other medical equipment, got it up and running again in time for the next trip to Haiti.

TEEN #2—THE BASKETBALL STAR

On the next trip, the two medical team members were a cardiologist (heart specialist) and an internist (general internal medicine doctor). They brought the usual potpourri of donated supplies, along with the now refurbished EKG machine, courtesy of Daniel and the robotics club. Although Daniel was not on this trip, the cardiologist's sixteen-year-old son Trevor was one of the volunteers. Tall, handsome, and athletic, Trevor was a star on his school's basketball team. The cardiologist's participation on the trip, as well as his son's, was something of a fluke. At home, the cardiologist had gone to watch one of Trevor's basketball games, but there was a mix-up in the schedule and Dad went to the wrong game. At that game, he ran into the aforementioned internist who had been on these Haiti trips in the past. The internist told the cardiologist about the missions, sparking the cardiologist's interest and prompting him to make the next trip and bring his son. The internist's teenage son would also be going on the trip.

Shortly after arrival, the physicians on the team were anxious to test the EKG machine to see if it still worked after the arduous trip to the remote clinic. It wasn't as easy as they'd hoped, though, because although they had a machine now, they realized they didn't have the lead wires necessary to attach the machine to a patient. They were about to give up on having a functioning EKG machine that trip, but thanks to the industrious and determined efforts of a nurse also on the volunteer team from the U.S., they were able to find the lead wires they needed.

The two teenage boys, Trevor and the son of the internist, were standing next to each other in the clinic when their physician fathers wanted to try out the machine for the first time. Neither boy was much interested in being the first "guinea pig" volunteer, but the cardiologist insisted it be his son so as not to impose on his colleague's son. They clipped the standard twelve lead wires to electrodes placed on Trevor's chest and turned on the machine. Indeed, it worked. But as soon as the strip of paper with the test results came out of the machine, a collective gasp filled the room—what they saw on the EKG test on this seemingly healthy young man was devastating. This strapping, athletic teen had a potentially lethal heart defect.

This was the very beginning of the trip, but his dad, the cardiologist, knew he had to get Trevor to a major medical facility. They carefully observed him until the first opportunity to return to the States, when he was admitted to a premier medical center. He was evaluated by the heart surgeon there, who told the family the boy needed urgent open-heart surgery to correct a life-threatening heart defect, probably present since birth but not detected until the serendipitous testing in this remote Haitian village with a patched-up EKG machine. The surgery was successful, and Trevor went on to become a nationally recognized high-school basketball player.

TEEN #3—THE MALNOURISHED ORPHAN

A few weeks after Trevor's lifesaving experience at the clinic, a fourteen-year-old girl named Betiane was brought to the same clinic by her aunt to see the current medical team, of which I was a part. As a pediatric specialist, I was the designated caregiver for most of the kids we saw during my volunteer trips to this clinic in Haiti. This young girl, in tattered clothes and appearing frightened, sat in my exam chair. She was extraordinarily thin and clearly malnourished.

Even more urgently, Betiane had such severe difficulty breathing she could not complete a sentence without gasping for air. I listened to her chest with my stethoscope and heard the loudest heart murmur I can ever remember hearing. A heart murmur is the sound blood makes when flowing through abnormal compartments or valves in the heart. I then knew she had heart disease, but did not know what type. Our EKG machine, the same machine that had been repaired by Daniel, our robotics club volunteer, and the same machine that saved the life of Trevor, our star basketball volunteer, confirmed our suspicions of severe heart disease as the cause of Betiane's breathing distress. At this point, we suspected she had rheumatic heart disease, a dread complication of a childhood strep infection (usually strep throat). Rheumatic heart disease is rarely seen in the United States any longer because of timely use of antibiotics for strep infections, but in the developing world and impoverished communities, rheumatic heart disease remains a significant and life-threatening problem. Betiane needed surgery if she had any hope of surviving—and surgery was an impossibility in this setting.

As if that wasn't enough, Betiane's aunt announced that because of her own dire poverty, she could no longer care for the child. We learned that the girl's mother had died, after which her aunt took over her care. The child's father was never involved. The aunt had tried her best but was now giving up for the sake of the girl who needed more than the aunt could possibly provide. Betiane's profound malnutrition was testimony to the aunt's desperate situation. As the aunt walked away from her niece forever, I left the examining room in tears for what this child was going through, trying to pull myself together for what we next needed to do. Betiane would surely die of malnutrition if the profound breathing distress from her heart disease didn't kill her first.

Struggling for breath, Betiane walked with us a mile to a nearby orphanage where we begged them to take the girl into their already overcrowded and overwhelmed facility. The orphanage had no medicines, but agreed to provide the girl with food and shelter to the best of their ability. I left feeling overwhelmed with sadness, fearing I would never see her again. With all our good intentions, there was nothing more we could do for this poor child.

POSTSCRIPT

But the story didn't end there for our teens. Through his dad (the cardiologist who was now part of the medical teams serving the Haiti clinic), Trevor heard of Betiane's grave situation. Having himself been saved by the clinic and its valiant, patched-up little EKG machine, he was tormented to think that it was only because of his good fortune, living in the United States and being able to afford the best medical care in the world, that he would survive and Betiane would not. So when it came time for his hospital discharge following open-heart surgery, Trevor's surgeon came in to say good-bye and asked if there was anything else the boy needed before going home. Yes there was, he said. Trevor told the surgeon about Betiane and asked if he would be willing to operate on her if a way could be found to bring her to the States and to this premier medical facility. Would the surgeon give Betiane the gift of life as he had for the cardiologist's son? The surgeon didn't hesitate a moment—of course he would!

Turns out getting the surgeon to agree was the easy part. Betiane had no papers, no documentation of who she was or where she was from, and no way to leave the country. The bureaucratic hornet's nest that was then unleashed rivaled any medical challenges we had faced in Haiti. Between the governments of Haiti and the United States, and even turf wars within the medical community in the U.S., one hurdle after another seemed to doom Betiane to never leaving Haiti for the lifesaving surgery awaiting her in the U.S.

Meanwhile, in the orphanage, Betiane's nutrition improved somewhat and, as a result, she was in a little less breathing distress. On a subsequent visit to the same rural village in Haiti, an immigration attorney and a school-teacher were now part of the volunteer group. They, along with the nurse practitioner clinic medical director, went to plead Betiane's case at the U.S. Embassy in Port-au-Prince. Faced with more stonewalling, a call was finally placed to a newly elected U.S. senator from the state where the surgery would be done. With the senator's help, and the tireless determination of these volunteer individuals over many months, Betiane was flown to the U.S. where she, too, had open-heart surgery by the same doctor who had cared for Trevor. The surgeon replaced a heart valve ravaged by her rheumatic heart disease and the procedure was a success. The heart failure that had caused her severe breathing problems was cured.

Following discharge from the hospital, Betiane continued her recovery for the next three months in the home of another one of our medical colleagues from the Haiti missions. She returned to the orphanage, where we visited her on each of our subsequent trips to Haiti. Betiane, now seventeen years old, is healthy, well-nourished and, to our eyes, has become the "Queen Bee" of her orphanage. She is very grateful for the life she has been given.

So, to sum up, a donated but broken EKG machine was repaired by a teenage volunteer on a medical mission to Haiti. That machine returned to Haiti and diagnosed severe congenital heart disease on another teen volunteer who was only there because his dad had gone to the wrong basketball game. This teen had no symptoms of a heart problem, but he may well have very soon thereafter become one of those tragic cases we read about—a young athlete who collapses on the playing field or basketball court and cannot be resuscitated. Instead, that young athlete survived thanks to major surgery and not only continued to excel in his sports career, but also paved the way for lifesaving surgery for another teen who otherwise had no chance of survival.

Three teens, who never met each other, saved each other's lives with the help of a miraculous little machine in a remote Haitian clinic. Today, the machine continues in use daily and is still the only EKG machine we've ever had there.

DATE OF EVENT: JANUARY 2013

An Impossible Delivery

Amanda Yeaton-Massey, MD
Kay Daniels, MD

When Karen walked into the emergency room she knew something was wrong. Since New Year's Eve she had felt an uncomfortable growth and had experienced some light vaginal bleeding, a rare occurrence as she had not had a period in five years. Her first thought was that this was another episode of vaginal bleeding from her *uterine fibroids* to add to her long list of previous emergency room visits for the same problem. Uterine fibroids are benign tumors of the uterus that can cause heavy and prolonged menstrual bleeding, with sometimes serious consequences. With this episode, as with some of her previous ones, her bleeding had gotten so heavy she could no longer manage it at home. A tall, fit woman of forty, Karen had undergone numerous treatments for her condition, including surgical removal and a procedure known as *uterine artery embolization* intended to cut off the blood supply to the fibroids. She was unsure what to attribute this bleeding episode to as she had only rare spotting in the years following the procedure.

Karen and her husband had been told that the lifesaving procedures to decrease the bleeding from her fibroids had likely rendered her infertile. While they had wanted children, they had made the decision to save Karen's life and had shifted the way they envisioned their family. Waiting patiently on her gurney for an ultrasound, she tried to quiet the nagging sense that something was different this time. She lay on her back in the dimly lit room with her exposed belly covered in the blob of blue gel used for the ultrasound test. A quiet fell over the room when the tech placed the probe over her abdomen to reveal not fibroids but a fetus. It moved. Its heart beat. It was a female and, as it turned out, had been growing inside Karen for almost seven months. As the ultrasound continued, the apparent cause of her bleeding was revealed: a *placenta previa*, an abnormally located placenta covering the opening to her cervix. She and her husband now took in the wonderful news that they would be parents and the terrifying news that the location of her placenta posed a threat to both Karen's life and that of their growing child.

Karen was quickly transferred to a hospital equipped with a neonatal intensive care unit that could care for her baby and a high-risk obstetric team that could care for her. The ultrasound was repeated once she was admitted to the second hospital and confirmed her seven-month pregnancy and the abnormal location of the placenta. This ultrasound, however, also demonstrated an area of the placenta that appeared to be invading into the wall of the uterus, a very dangerous condition known as *placenta accreta*. While a placenta previa typically requires delivery by caesarean section near the completion of the pregnancy (as long as bleeding can be controlled prior to that), a placenta accreta typically requires immediate delivery by caesarean section followed by a hysterectomy (complete removal of the uterus). Thankfully, Karen's bleeding stopped and she had a few days to absorb some of this life-changing information.

I was in my second year as a resident on the high-risk obstetrics service and had the pleasure of seeing Karen and her husband daily on rounds. I watched as they gracefully came to terms with the news of her pregnancy along with the potentially life-threatening complications. Karen was a vivacious woman who would have much preferred being on a hiking trail than in a hospital and she yearned to return to her home and friends. She walked the halls every day to get out of her room and develop some semblance of normalcy. I would visit with Karen and her husband on these walks and listen to stories of their community banding together to get their home ready for their baby. They shared with me that their little girl would be named after Karen's late mother-in-law. The baby was becoming more real by the day and the team could tell these two would be incredible parents. We hoped, though, that we would all have a chance to wait a few weeks to meet their little girl, who needed more time to grow and develop inside her mother.

After two relatively quiet weeks in the hospital where she was carefully being monitored, Karen developed sudden, excruciating abdominal pain and contractions. She was rushed to the ultrasound suite for evaluation where, to the shock of everyone in the room, her fetus was noted to be freely floating outside of her uterus, in her abdomen, which was full of what was likely amniotic fluid. Her uterus had ruptured, expelling the baby, and now her baby was at imminent risk of separation from its uterine lifeline; the fetus and umbilical cord would likely tear away from the uterus at any moment. Without immediate delivery the infant could die from lack of oxygen, and Karen could die from massive bleeding.

Minutes after receiving this catastrophic news, the team was wheeling Karen from the ultrasound suite to the operating room. My heart pounded as I held her hand and tried to reassure her and her husband that we would do everything we could to save Karen and their infant. With anesthesia at the head, her nurse on the left and me on the right we were an unlikely sight as we raced the unwieldy gurney and IV pole down the hall. As our convoy entered the doors to the operating suite we were pointed down the hall to the room being prepared for her. There was a palpable sense of urgency as word of Karen's extraordinary circumstances preceded her.

Karen was transferred to the operating table, as the staff got ready for an emergency surgery and the pediatrics team readied for the arrival of her premature baby. Every second counted, and the teams worked in concert to expedite this critical delivery. We worked against the sickening knowledge that such a large uterine rupture was unlikely to be survivable for her baby and, even if survivable, unlikelier still to result in a child who was neurologically intact. A baby's brain function depends on sufficient oxygen being delivered through an intact and in-place umbilical cord connected to the placenta. As soon as the surgical drapes were placed to frame Karen's abdomen, an incision was made from her pubic bone to beneath her breasts, revealing a free-floating infant with only its head remaining inside the uterus. The rest of the baby's body protruded into the abdominal cavity through the massive tear in the uterus. The cord was clamped and cut and the baby girl was handed off to awaiting pediatricians, floppy but miraculously very much alive.

No one could believe it but the placenta accreta, which now posed an imminent threat to Karen's life, had saved her baby with its tenacious grip on the uterus in spite of the rupture. The placenta had deeply invaded the wall of the uterus, tightly anchoring itself. Under just about any other circumstance with a uterine rupture of this size, the placenta would have ripped completely away from the uterus, leaving the fetus floating helplessly in the abdominal cavity, without blood supply or oxygen. Invasion of the placenta into the uterus is a dreaded obstetric complication, one typically seen with prior caesarean section scars. It is associated with massive blood loss and usually requires removal of the uterus with the placenta after delivery of the infant to save the mother's life. In Karen's case she had no caesarean scar on her uterus, only the procedures to remove her fibroids and decrease blood supply. The likelihood of her having a placenta accreta was low and in this case this dangerous abnormal placental growth was the only thing that saved her infant's life. The baby was, as it turned out, saved by the very placental abnormality that initially announced her presence and put her mother's life at risk. One life-threatening complication of pregnancy, the placenta accreta, rescued both mother and baby from another life-threatening complication of pregnancy, a ruptured uterus.

Incredibly, Karen underwent an uncomplicated hysterectomy to remove both her uterus and the invasive placenta. In spite of massive blood loss, she was moved from the intensive care unit to the regular postpartum floor the day after her surgery. Now, more than a year-and-a-half later, Karen is completely recovered from her ordeal and joyously watching her absolutely perfect baby girl thrive as she discovers the world around her.

Periodically Karen will send pictures of her miracle baby. They serve as moving reminders that sometimes everything conspires to make the impossible possible.

DATE OF EVENT: EARLY 2000s

Exploding Blood Cells

Philip L. Glick, MD, MBA

A fourteen-year-old boy from a dairy farm in the rural part of the Northeast was admitted to our intensive care unit (ICU) with a serious condition called *hemolytic uremic syndrome* (HUS). This illness is usually caused by certain types of bacteria in food, but has also been linked to swimming in contaminated lake water, which was the suspected source in this child's case. HUS begins with the gradual bursting of red blood cells, causing anemia. The debris from the burst cells can clog the kidneys and cause them to fail. Other organs of the body are less commonly affected. The prognosis for the typical case of HUS in a child is excellent. However this was, in no way, a typical case.

This boy developed kidney failure, the most common serious complication of the disease; however, he was quite stable for several days in the ICU. Our surgical service was consulted because of the possible need for dialysis should his kidney function deteriorate further. Dialysis involves hooking up a filtering machine to the patient's blood vessels through a catheter tube and running the patient's entire blood circulation through the machine to clear the toxins, returning "clean" blood back to the patient. Removing toxins is a normal function of the kidneys, but with kidney failure, toxins accumulate and, without dialysis, these can be very dangerous.

After another stable day, the child's kidney function gradually deteriorated further and we made the decision to mobilize the surgical team and take him to the operating room at 12:30 AM for placement of a dialysis catheter, rather than waiting until a more "normal" hour and risking further decline in his kidney function. He remained quite stable as we rolled him in, and we anticipated a very routine procedure. As we were obtaining consent for surgery from the parents, the boy's heart monitor suddenly showed that he had developed a very abnormal heartbeat pattern, the type caused by excessive levels of potassium in the blood. There could be only one explanation for such high levels of potassium so suddenly: a massive explosion of the child's red blood cells (which contain high levels of potassium). Whereas his HUS had caused a more gradual destruction of blood cells up until that point, the illness now had taken a potentially lethal turn with simultaneous bursting of millions of blood cells.

As a result of the destruction of so many red blood cells all at once, there weren't enough left to sufficiently carry oxygen to the vital parts of the body, including the brain. This profound anemia forced the child's heart to overwork trying to get too few cells to too many places in the body. Adding to the crisis was the excessive potassium from the burst cells. Potassium, in high levels, is extremely toxic to the heart. The child suddenly went into cardiac arrest on the operating room table, and we instantly began cardiopulmonary resuscitation (CPR). But we knew this child would very likely die unless we did something dramatic—*immediately*—to save his heart and brain.

There was only one "something" that might work: an invasive and potentially dangerous technique called *extracorporeal membrane oxygenation*, or ECMO. ECMO does for the heart and lungs what dialysis does for the kidneys. It siphons all the blood from the body into a machine that puts oxygen into the blood and removes carbon dioxide, as a normally functioning heart and the lungs do with each breath we take. This child's failed heart was unable to get sufficient blood to his lungs, and ECMO was our only option.

While the team was still performing CPR, I ran out to find the parents and explain, as quickly and completely as I could, how our plans for a routine dialysis catheter insertion had changed to an emergent lifesaving and high-risk ECMO procedure. I cautioned the boy's parents that ECMO itself can cause brain damage because of the removal and replacement of the child's entire blood pool, the blood thinners required to keep the blood flowing smoothly through the machine, and the potential disruptions of blood flow to the brain that any step of the procedure can cause.

There are some miracles that seem to occur because circumstances are just right for a miracle, a perfect "alignment of the stars" that allows for an astonishing outcome. Heart failure as a complication of HUS is very rare and often fatal. Had this child's massive explosion of red blood cells occurred at home, in an ambulance, in a small community hospital, or even in a different part of our tertiary care children's hospital, he would likely have died. Instead, his life-threatening, instantaneous deterioration developed before our eyes, on the operating room table, as we were preparing him for a much more routine surgical procedure. The ICU team with an ECMO machine was only a few steps away, the veins into which we were going to have to insert the ECMO catheters had already been scrubbed with iodine in preparation for the dialysis catheter insertion, and the surgical team was already in place in the wee early hours of the morning. It was as if this boy's body "waited for the right minute" to give out.

We finished the procedure at 3:00 AM and brought the child to the ICU. At 6:30 AM, as my team made rounds, we found him awake and alert, but I was a little concerned that he might have been somewhat dulled in his responses to my questions. Had his cardiac arrest, prolonged CPR, or ECMO caused neurologic damage? At 8:30 that morning, I found Mom at the bedside and asked her what she thought of his condition—specifically, his speech, thought processes, level of awareness, etc. She couldn't figure out what I was concerned about—he's perfect, she said, completely normal.

"Never was a rocket scientist, never will be, but he's exactly who he was before; my boy, the love of my life!" With a big hug and tears in both of our eyes she said, "Thank you, Dr. Glick, and thank your team. Bless you!"

She and I couldn't have been more grateful for the miracle of this boy's extraordinary timing.

DATE OF EVENT: APRIL 2015

Right Where She Needed to Be

Matthew Old, MD

As a head and neck cancer surgeon, my patients are typically referred to me by physicians of many different specialties; patients don't typically seek me out on their own. One day, however, a young woman working at our cancer hospital stopped me in the hallway and asked me for my opinion about her symptoms. This self-referral could not have been more appropriate or timely, and it may well have saved her life.

Elli was a college freshman interning at our cancer center. Her position was not initially supposed to be on our surgery floor, but just before starting her job she was reassigned here. I had spoken with Elli many times on the phone through her work as a liaison with the families of our patients, but I had never before met her face-to-face.

Elli told me an incredible story of symptoms lasting more than five years: dizziness, lightheadedness, intermittent face swelling, and periods of vision and hearing "blackouts." She saw numerous doctors over that long period of time, each with a different, but reassuring, theory about what was causing her symptoms: iron deficiency, hormone changes, anxiety, recurring upper respiratory infections, and chronic tonsillitis. She received antibiotics, iron pills, and steroids to treat a variety of possible ailments suggested by the doctors. She even had her tonsils taken out. Nothing helped. She had to give up high school basketball because it made the symptoms worse, but then they began occurring during normal daily activities as well. She would fall asleep with her head to the side and wake up with stroke-like symptoms—imbalance, dizziness, nausea, and weakness. She told me she suspected something bad was happening, and then was sure of it when she felt a lump in her neck.

When I examined Elli's mouth, I was very disturbed to find that the back of her throat wasn't symmetric. The tissues on one side of her throat were displaced off to the side and bulging into her neck space. I ordered a CAT scan (a special kind of X-ray) and what we saw floored us—a large, baseball-size tumor at the base of her skull was totally surrounding her right carotid artery. One nerve to her tongue and voice box was already compromised by the tumor, paralyzing half of her tongue and one of her vocal cords. Carotid arteries, one on each side of the neck, provide the major source of blood, and therefore oxygen, to our brains. Elli's tumor was so large it was not only stealing blood from her carotid artery, but also compressing the artery itself. Through a series of scans I determined the tumor was cutting off the blood flow to her brain, causing all of her symptoms for the past several years. If it continued to grow, she would almost certainly have a stroke and, possibly, lose her life. When I informed Elli about the tumor, she said she was relieved she had an answer to everything she was experiencing and that she was not "crazy" and didn't have an anxiety disorder. On the other hand, her family was devastated, learning that suddenly her life was in a precarious balance, particularly with what she was about to face.

Our team concluded the tumor had to be removed—but the surgery we would need to perform was very complicated and risky, and could itself cause a stroke. To make matters worse, it was not only the carotid artery that was at risk due to the tumor—the nerves controlling her face, tongue, throat, and voice box were also at risk due to the location of the tumor. These are rare surgeries but I had training in them and had performed them previously, so I was confident and optimistic. However, due to the high stakes and severity of her symptoms, it was nerve-racking and stressful for all of us.

What ensued next is among the finest examples of collaborative surgery I have ever been privileged to be a part of. It took seventeen hours for our extraordinary team of three different surgeons to dissect, pry apart, tease away, and finally remove the entire tumor from Elli's neck and base of skull. The surgery was harrowing; if we tilted her head to one side or the other, her vital signs would change—blood pressure and pulse would drop—because we were altering the blood flow to her brain through her severely narrowed carotid artery. During the procedure we realized we couldn't save the nerves to her vocal cords and tongue. We successfully preserved her hearing and the nerves to her face so she wouldn't have a droop. Even after surgery, we still held our breath as we noticed her lower left leg was paralyzed—but, thankfully, it is slowly recovering. Elli was left with a slightly raspy voice, weakness on the right side of her tongue, and a temporary limp. But she survived with intact hearing, no facial droop and, most importantly, without suffering a major stroke or other devastating complication. We were all relieved she pulled through it, but I credit this mostly to her resolve and determination to overcome obstacles.

To look at her today, you would have no idea what Elli has been through. Her recovery should have taken more than a year, but she returned to work two months after surgery to a surprise standing ovation from the entire staff of the surgery floor. She now uses her experiences to help our other hospitalized patients and families get through difficult times dealing with cancer and surgery. Not long after, Elli returned to college, a pre-med major, hoping to be a children's cancer doctor someday.

We now know Elli's tumor was a *vagal paraganglioma*, a very rare tumor occurring in less than one in every five million people. She, of course, had no way of knowing she had a rare paraganglioma when she stopped me in the hallway. She had heard about lymphomas, a different kind of tumor that can occur in the neck, and she was worried that's what she had. Elli also had no way of knowing that during my training as a head and neck surgeon, my mentor was an expert in this very type of highly specialized paraganglioma surgery and taught me to become expert in that procedure as well.

There are a lot of other hospitals in town where Elli could have worked. In our hospital, there are many doctors on many different floors including many even on our surgical floor—innumerable other white-coated colleagues Elli could have asked for help. But Elli chose to work in our hospital where she asked me. Only because I worked on the same floor as she did—the floor she had been switched to at the last minute before starting her internship. As a result, an almost certain stroke was prevented just in time, and her life may have been saved as well.

Call this a case of good luck: being right where she needed to be, right when she needed to be there; doing the right job, with all the right people working beside her. Or call it serendipity, the alignment of all the stars to result in a wonderful outcome. Or call it a miracle. She and her family do, and so do I.

DATE OF EVENT:1999

When Sister Bernie Prays for You

Claudette Dalton, MD

I met Sister Bernie Kenny in the late 1990s when I organized a medical team from our university medical center to go to the mountains of southwest Virginia to help with a weekend dental and medical clinic. Sister Bernie is a Catholic nun who ran an organization called the St. Mary's Health Wagon. This group of dedicated nurses drove around the Appalachian region near the town of Wise, in southwestern Virginia, to provide basic medical and follow-up care to the residents of the area. Geographically, this area is the "tail" of Virginia, sitting between West Virginia, Tennessee, and Kentucky. Coal mining, logging, and railroads are the main industries, but these are largely played out and dwindling along with the region. Consequently, most of the remaining population is uninsured, unemployed, and poor. They also have some of the highest rates of chronic diseases, cancer, and drug abuse in the state.

Sister Bernie also knew that there was almost no dental care in this area. So she asked a nonprofit organization called Remote Area Medical (RAM) clinic to help provide a free, once-a-year dental clinic. RAM, based in Knoxville, Tennessee, worked with the Virginia Dental Association to provide dental care over a hot summer weekend in an unused airplane hangar at the Lonesome Pine Airport just outside of Wise. Unfortunately, many of the patients were too ill with diabetes, hypertension, or heart disease to safely have dental work done. So, in planning for the next year, Sister Bernie called me to put together a medical team to complement the dental efforts.

I'm proud to say we had no trouble finding medical volunteers to spend a steamy, muddy July weekend in a remote, deserted airplane hangar more than six hours away from my home base in Charlottesville. The generosity of this extraordinary group of doctors and nurses from all over Virginia and beyond has become legendary and their work continues each summer now for the past sixteen years. But that first year, I had no idea what supplies and services we would need, where we would house and feed the team, how we would transport them and how we would follow up on patients. In the midst of this planning chaos, I got another call from Sister Bernie, now just two weeks before the event.

"Do you know," she asked, "where we could get a mammogram van for the event?"

I replied that, as an anesthesiologist, I knew nothing about mammogram vans and I didn't think I had the time or expertise to help her. We were in enough tumult just trying to get a medical team to Wise.

"But we have women scheduled to have mammograms," she said. She explained that the van she had borrowed in the past for her traveling Health Wagon program was sold to someone who wouldn't let her use it. I repeated my total inability to be of any possible help to her, especially at this late date. Mammogram vans don't just grow on trees.

"We need a van. These women have masses and need films," she insisted. As I opened my mouth to restate my position, she said, "I'm praying for you!" and she hung up the phone. I was completely dumbfounded!

I called the mammogram radiologist at my institution who confirmed we had no van and suggested calling another medical school, this one in Richmond. The Richmond school suggested the military. When I finally found who to call at military bases in Virginia, none of them could help. Finally, after dozens of random calls to community clinics, someone said there was an old van on blocks (no wheels) in Mount Rogers—some four hours away from us. By now, it was four days until we were to leave for the clinic in the mountains.

Now the miracles started to flow. The Mount Rogers Health District said yes, they had an old van, but it was not accredited and the equipment had not been used in years. But they would put tires on it and drive it to our university medical center. Our head mammography radiologist managed to get it refurbished and accredited—in forty-eight hours. Two days to refurbish a neglected, outdated van and accredit the neglected, outdated mammography equipment! I never asked how she did it and I never will ask. And two days before we went, I was coincidentally scheduled for my own mammogram at our medical center. The techs who took care of me offered, out of the clear blue, to go to Wise with me two days later to run the machinery and perform the mammograms!

Somehow, we managed to get the van and all the volunteers to the abandoned mountain airport hangar. The ancient machinery worked fine through Friday and Saturday, finally giving out on Sunday morning, but not before thirty women and a couple of men with breast lumps had their mammograms. Because of this confluence of small miracles to make one giant one, four women and one man with early breast cancer were detected and successfully treated. All did well.

The miracles didn't stop with that one clinic. As a result of our experience and Sister Bernie's persistence, our university medical center bought the van, completely updated it with new mammography equipment, and drove it all around the state serving underprivileged patients for three more years. That was so successful, they bought a new, better van and used that for another four to five years. They are now on their third van with state-of-the-art equipment. Countless lives have been saved by those vans.

For me, the moral of this story is that if Sister Bernie prays for you, shut up and get busy, because the miracles are gonna happen—and they're gonna happen fast.

DATE OF EVENT: 2005

He Was Lucky He Had AIDS

Mark F. Cotton, MMed (Paed), PhD

Barbara Laughton, MBChB, DCH, MSc

We had been planning this study since 2001, developing methods for conducting a treatment trial in babies born with *HIV* (*human immunodeficiency virus*) infection, the virus that causes *AIDS* (*acquired immune deficiency syndrome*). The study was to evaluate which approach to treating these babies was most effective—early (soon after birth) therapy for a limited time, versus deferring therapy until the signs and symptoms of AIDS develop. The latter approach was our standard at the time. You might ask, "Isn't earlier therapy always better?" Well, not always. It's possible that the side effects of medicines could make earlier therapy in younger babies more dangerous. Or maybe treating before the signs and symptoms of AIDS develop would be less effective than hitting the infection hard as soon as symptoms occurred.

But there was also another overriding issue—South Africa, where we care for babies with AIDS, has an impoverished public sector with very limited resources. Patients able to pay for expensive treatments could get them, but most patients were dependent on government clinics and resources. A limited course of therapy might be more *cost*-effective and consume fewer resources than long-term treatment started once symptoms began. And if it was more cost-effective, we could treat more children. But if we found that early therapy was more effective, could we then stop it after a limited amount of time and still see benefit? We didn't know. If not, most patients would only improve for the time they were on medicine, and when the funds for the medicine ran out, they would worsen and could die. If we started treatment only after signs of the disease began, perhaps the same limited course of medicine would allow survival to an older age. The answers weren't clear to us at all, hence the research study.

The study finally began in 2005, and it showed that early therapy, even for a limited time, gave better results for these babies. That was a very important finding and helped us plan treatment for tens of thousands of HIV-infected babies in Africa, for whom our resources were limited and had to be used judiciously.

But that wasn't the miracle.

One of the devastating effects of AIDS in babies is impairment of brain function. As part of the study at our clinical trial site in Cape Town, we sought to determine the neuro-developmental impacts of the two different study approaches (early versus deferred treatment): how did the babies do in their childhood development: their ability to move around (locomotor skills) and coordinate precision movements (fine motor skills); interactions with their environment (personal-social skills); hearing and language development; hand-eye coordination, and their ability to think and reason. Once again, our study found early therapy had a better outcome on babies' brains than waiting for signs and symptoms of AIDS to occur before beginning treatment. That reinforced our commitment to early therapy.

But that still wasn't the miracle.

The miracle is the story of one little HIV-infected baby in this large and complicated research study. This little boy, Isaiah (not his real name), had a bigger head than normal but otherwise was well when he entered our AIDS treatment study. However, he started having seizures, and the vigilant study doctor ordered a brain scan, which showed unusual features suggesting this baby had something called an *inborn error of metabolism*, or IEM. An IEM means the chemical systems usually responsible for processing the food we eat and generating the energy and building blocks we need to survive have gone awry. In much of the Western world, especially now, routine screening of all newborns for inborn errors is conducted. That's because recognizing these defects early in life, before the ravages of the mistaken chemical reactions can take place, can save babies' lives and protect their brains. Mental retardation and severe developmental delays are the usual outcomes of babies who survive IEMs. But in South Africa at the time, and in much of the underdeveloped world still today, the luxury of screening for rare diseases doesn't exist. Babies in South Africa in 2005 were not screened for IEMs. (Unfortunately, that remains true as we are writing this in 2015.) Only this baby was screened, because he had HIV infection and was in our AIDS research study, where he was noticed to have abnormal features suggesting an IEM.

AIDS and IEMs are unrelated to each other—one doesn't cause or predispose to the other. Both damage babies' brains, but in different ways. It turned out this baby had both. Isaiah was tested and discovered to have an IEM called *glutaric aciduria type 1*. This is a treatable disease, but only if it's recognized early. In South Africa, it's rarely if ever recognized early. Untreated, it causes toxic buildup of chemicals in the brain, causing developmental delay, seizures, abnormal muscle tone, and movement disorders that resemble cerebral palsy. Treatment is actually easy and relatively cheap: mostly nutritional, avoiding foods containing chemicals that cannot be processed correctly because of the defect, and supplementing with other foods to provide adequate nutrition. This is especially important at times of metabolic stress such as during fevers. When glutaric aciduria type 1 is treated early, the results are very favorable.

Isaiah was treated early for both his HIV infection and for his IEM. His AIDS was treated with three effective medicines provided for him early in his life as part of the research trial. His inborn error was also treated early, but only because he was "lucky" enough to be infected with the virus that causes AIDS and to have been noticed to have a large head and seizures during his evaluation for the AIDS study. Isaiah did well on both counts, controlling his AIDS and his IEM.

A study published in 2010 reviewed the outcomes of more than a dozen kids diagnosed with glutaric aciduria type 1 in South Africa once reliable testing became widely available around 2008. All but one of those babies who, like Isaiah, was by chance diagnosed early (not as part of an AIDS trial, but as part of a different research trial), were devastated by the defect. We believe Isaiah and that other baby are the only children born in Africa with this IEM prior to 2008 who turned out neurologically normal.

Yes, Isaiah was lucky he was infected with the AIDS virus.

For more information about the research on the best approach to therapy in South African babies born with AIDS, see:

MF Cotton, A Violari, K Otwombe, et al. Early time-limited antiretroviral therapy versus deferred therapy in South African infants infected with HIV: results from the children with HIV early antiretroviral (CHER) randomised trial. *Lancet* 2013; 382: 1555–63.

B Laughton, M Cornell, D Grove, et al. Early antiretroviral therapy improves neurodevelopmental outcomes in infants. *AIDS.* 2012 Aug 24; 26 (13): 1685–90.

For more information on glutaric aciduria type 1 in South African children, see:

G van der Watt, E Owen, P Berman, et al. Glutaric aciduria type 1 in South Africa—high incidence of glutaryl-CoA dehydrogenase deficiency in black South Africans. *Molecular Genetics and Metabolism* 101: 2010. 178–182.

2

Impossible Cures

There is one situation where doctors are thrilled to be proven wrong—when we have told patients and families that recovery was impossible, only to discover, in time, that things turned out miraculously better than we expected. Not every dire diagnosis follows its expected course, and not every inevitablity is inevitable, giving reason for hope to those receiving the diagnosis—and to those of us giving it.

This chapter includes stories of astonishing cures from cancer, severe infections, and mysterious illnesses for which no cause could be found. The patients described in these essays were expected by their doctors to die or suffer permanent disability, yet all of them defied those expectations. To this day, we don't know how.

A Gift to Others Becomes a Miracle for Their Child

Rodney E. Willoughby, MD

Fifteen-year-old Jeanna was sitting in church with her mother when parishioners were startled from their worship by a bat that started swooping around overhead. Bats are nocturnal creatures, and this one was likely attempting to get back outside when a man swatted it to the ground. Jeanna loved animals (except spiders) and wanted to help the bat, so she picked it up by the wing tips to release it outside. As she set it free, however, the bat bit her left index finger.

Back at home, Jeanna's mother put peroxide on the wound. Thinking that would be enough to prevent an infection, nobody talked to a doctor. One month later, Jeanna was playing in a volleyball tournament but felt washed out. She developed fever and double vision, and she became less alert. She was admitted to the hospital on a weekend, and shortly thereafter began to have involuntary jerking of her left arm.

Her regular pediatrician had the weekend off, but he visited her in the hospital that Monday. She was rapidly worsening, so he arranged for transport to our university hospital ninety minutes away, where she could be seen by all the appropriate specialists. He then did what all good doctors do when things aren't going as expected—he took another history of her illness in case the other doctors had missed some key piece of information. He was the first to learn about the bat bite that had occurred a month earlier, so he called our transport physician with this new information. The transport physician, in turn, called me from the command center to ask whether we should consider rabies. Rabies is a lethal virus infection usually transmitted by bites or other contact with infected animals. Despite practicing as an infectious diseases doctor for twenty years, I had never seen a patient with rabies, but I did know rabies patients always died. *Always.* I suggested that the transport team use personal protective equipment just in case, to avoid the need for rabies shots. I organized the hospital tests to quickly exclude rabies, a diagnosis I doubted, so we could get on with treating whatever it was she "really" had. We sent the rabies tests off that same day to the Centers for Disease Control and Prevention (CDC) in Atlanta, expecting an answer late the next day.

That night, Jeanna started salivating profusely, requiring insertion of a tube into her windpipe and connected to a machine to support her breathing. Her disease course began to sound more and more like rabies, so I did some reading in between seeing other patients. The medical literature discussed the fact that there was no actual damage to the brain despite the very violent brain activity triggered in the clinical disease we call rabies. I came across a paper from the world-famous Pasteur Institute in Paris. (Louis Pasteur invented milk pasteurization, and also the rabies vaccine in the 1880s. Rabies vaccine protects people who have been exposed to rabies, but does not treat patients like Jeanna who are already infected.) That article used ketamine, a general anesthetic, with good effect against experimental rabies in rats. Because rabies was so medically violent, causing brain hyperactivity capable of stopping the heart in an instant, it seemed wise to suppress brain function to avoid this complication. Ketamine seemed to be the right drug to use for general anesthesia during rabies, although it had never been tried before in humans.

Several articles in the medical literature described "near misses"—patients who almost survived but died of complications attributed to medical care. These near-miss patients appeared to have cleared the rabies virus from their bodies by themselves after one to two weeks. So I decided to use ketamine anesthesia on Jeanna in hopes of protecting her brain until her own body could clear the virus by itself, in a week or two.

The idea seemed simple—really, too simple. Why hadn't it been tried before? Most made-up-on-the-spot medical treatments cause grievous harm. When the diagnosis of rabies was confirmed by the CDC that next afternoon, we assembled seven experts in brain diseases, infections, and critical care. I proposed my idea to the physicians, intending to stop right there if any of my experts thought our plan would cause harm. We agreed to offer our strategy to Jeanna's family as the third of three options. The first option was conventional care, which had never worked in rabies; the second option was hospice care to speed her passing without pain or suffering.

Her parents understood the terminal diagnosis for Jeanna, and listened to our options of standard or hospice care. They asked for another option. We explained our theory that had never been tried before, even in animals other than rats. To my great surprise, they selected the third option, an untested experiment, "So that maybe we might learn something to save the next child." We were greatly humbled by this selfless gesture from Jeanna's parents who, despite being distraught over their daughter's condition, were thinking ahead for others.

We immediately sedated Jeanna with ketamine to the point of coma, and planned to wait and observe for a week. While I was writing the plan for her care, a very pleasant priest in civilian clothes arrived by her door and asked if he could pray over her. I helped him into appropriate protective clothing: a gown, mask, gloves, shoe covering, and head covering. A little while later he thanked me and went on his way. Still writing in her medical record twenty minutes later, I was approached by another priest who identified himself as the pastor of the church where she had been bitten. He asked if he could pray over her. I responded in jest that somebody just had, but that we could use all the prayers we could assemble. He then asked who had been by earlier, and one of the nurses responded, "Oh, Bishop Dolan."

Rather than the tumultuous and terrifying neurologic and other organ system failures caused by the severe brain dysfunction characteristic of most patients dying of rabies, the days passed uneventfully for Jeanna. After a week, we repeated our studies on rabies to confirm that her immune response to rabies had developed. It had, so we stopped her sedation.

Her brain wave tests immediately improved, and her pupils constricted to light, a good sign, but nothing else worked. She was fully paralyzed and showed no response to touch or voice. I was devastated, thinking that I had created a situation worse than death. This is called being "locked in," meaning you are aware and thinking, but cannot move and are restricted to communication by eye blinks. Two days later, she appeared no better. Then another doctor caring for Jeanna told me she had detected leg jerks when tapping her knees with a reflex hammer. I rushed to Jeanna's bed and indeed the reflexes were there! Every day after that, Jeanna made a new step toward her eventual recovery. She improved at a pace far faster than I've ever encountered with other brain infections.

Still, her recovery was long, hard work. She had to come back from full paralysis, learning to walk, talk, and eat all over again. Remarkably, she caught up with her high school studies with a tutor over the summer months, and started school with her same classmates that fall. Four years later, she was the first in her family to graduate from college. Today, Jeanna is indistinguishable from anyone else you might see on the street. She still loves animals and is an advocate for bat conservation. She is due to be married this next fall.

Jeanna was the first patient ever to survive rabies infection. Modified versions of the therapy we used for Jeanna have since been used for other patients with rabies, as Jeanna's parents had hoped when they courageously and generously chose "option three," and have resulted in additional cures. Was it her medical treatment or the power of prayer that was behind her survival? Some things we may never know. We do know that by releasing Jeanna for the benefit of others, her parents got her back.

Four and a half years later, on February 23, 2009, Bishop Dolan, who had come in to pray for Jeanna as our experimental therapy was just getting underway, was named Archbishop of New York by Pope Benedict XVI. His Eminence, Timothy Michael Cardinal Dolan, was installed in the archdiocese on April 15, 2009.

DATE OF EVENT: 1985

The First and Still the Most Miraculous

Harley A. Rotbart, MD

I was in the final month of my three-year fellowship in Pediatric Infectious Diseases when I was called to see Jonathan, a two-year-old former premature baby who couldn't shake his pneumonia. It had started out looking like a routine case of benign winter viral lung infection, a common problem in young children, especially former premature babies. But instead of the typical week or two course of those infections, Jonathan's pneumonia lingered for months, well into the spring. He initially required supplemental oxygen given through a tube in his nose. This should have been just a temporary treatment until his lungs healed. But whenever his doctors tried to "wean" Jonathan from the oxygen, he developed breathing distress, his lips turned blue, and the oxygen levels in his blood dropped.

When I was asked to evaluate Jonathan for the cause of this persistent lung disease, my first thought was his doctors had called the wrong specialist. Infections don't often cause chronic (long-lasting) lung disease in children. Before walking into his room for the first time, I reviewed in my head all the "usual suspects" for this type of problem. Cystic fibrosis, perhaps, or maybe an allergic form of pneumonia. I wondered if this could be an unusual appearance of asthma. Or, having been a premature baby, Jonathan might have a condition called *bronchopulmonary dysplasia*, a form of lung scarring resulting from treatment of immature lungs in babies born too early. None of those are due to infections, though, and I predicted my involvement with Jonathan's case would be short-lived. There were a few rare infections I would have to investigate—fungus infections unique to certain parts of the country or elsewhere in the world, for example. I would have to ask Jonathan's mother about their travel history. Pertussis, or whooping cough, can cause a persistent cough, but is preventable by vaccines. Of course, I would ask about Jonathan's immunization history.

After taking a careful history from Jonathan's mother, doing a thorough physical examination, and reviewing all of his X-rays, I was almost certain this was not an infection—at least not one I had seen or read about before. I discussed Jonathan's case with my infectious diseases attending (supervising) physician and presented Jonathan's story to our weekly infectious diseases meeting, where all of our colleagues from around the city met to review interesting and puzzling cases. We agreed on a panel of tests to perform to rule out infection as the cause of Jonathan's illness. During that next week, we tested Jonathan for all of the germs suggested as possibilities by the experts at the citywide conference. All the tests were negative. Our only remaining option for finding a cause and being able to get Jonathan off oxygen and back to a healthy toddler's life was a lung biopsy. The decision to do a lung biopsy is never taken lightly—it requires general anesthesia and surgery, both of which come with their own risks in addition to those associated with cutting out a piece of lung tissue. Jonathan's mother agreed with our recommendation for a lung biopsy, and Jonathan tolerated the procedure well and had no complications.

Four days later, the biopsy results came back. The diagnosis was one I had never heard of, nor had anyone else on our team: *lymphocytic interstitial pneumonia*, or LIP.

✧ ✧ ✧

I want to take a step back now for context. Jonathan's biopsy was performed in the summer of 1985. The first cases of *AIDS* (*acquired immune deficiency syndrome*) in gay men had been reported in the early 1980s in New York and San Francisco. The cause of AIDS was still being debated—most suspected an infection, but not everyone agreed. What kind of infection it might be was completely unknown. In December 1982, the first suspected case of AIDS acquired by blood transfusion occurred in California. In March 1983, the United States Public Health Service (USPHS) issued a warning that individuals in high-risk groups should not donate blood. In December 1984, a thirteen-year-old Indiana boy named Ryan White was diagnosed with AIDS. Ryan was born with hemophilia, an abnormal blood condition that causes episodes of severe bleeding; treatment for those bleeding episodes requires transfusion of blood products. After Ryan's diagnosis, he received national attention because of the community fear and panic he created simply by attempting to attend school. He and his mother helped educate the nation about AIDS. Tragically, Ryan died of the infection in 1990.

The first approved screening test for the AIDS virus (*HIV, human immunodeficiency virus*) in blood products wasn't approved until 1985. My patient, Jonathan, was born on March 19, 1983, simultaneously with the USPHS warnings about high-risk blood donors. As a tiny premature baby, he required numerous blood transfusions from donors who had given blood prior to the warnings. There wouldn't be an approved test for screening blood products for another two years.

✧ ✧ ✧

When the biopsy results showing LIP came back, we were stumped. What is LIP? This was in an era before the Internet, before Google. But as infectious diseases specialists, we knew a lot about the emerging AIDS epidemic on the coasts from the exploding medical literature on the topic, as well as from the hyperbolic media coverage the disease was receiving. We had never had a child with AIDS in Colorado. I called a colleague who had treated the first two adult patients with AIDS in the state and asked if he had heard of LIP. He hadn't seen it yet in any of his patients, but knew of adult patients in San Francisco who had the condition. He put us in touch with one of those experts, and we sent the slides from Jonathan's lung biopsy to him. Another two weeks went by before we heard that, indeed, Jonathan had "classic LIP," and the most likely cause was AIDS, acquired from the transfusions he received as a baby.

This was devastating news to Jonathan's mother and to us. That same summer, 1985, actor Rock Hudson publicly disclosed he had AIDS before his death from the infection. AIDS was now a household word and a widespread worry. We and Jonathan's mother and the rest of the reading world all knew AIDS was a fatal diagnosis. There were no known survivors of the disease at that point. The only treatment we had was for the complications of AIDS, not for AIDS itself. AIDS medicines weren't approved for use in adults until 1987 and not approved for use in children until 1990, the year Ryan White died. Jonathan was the first child with AIDS in Colorado, and one of the very first in the United States. Jonathan was infected with the AIDS virus as a premature baby in 1983, first diagnosed with AIDS in 1985, and then went untreated for years until the first medicine became available. Based on everything we knew then, and everything we know even now, there was absolutely no chance of survival. *None.*

We followed Jonathan in our infectious diseases and hematology clinics for several years after that, waiting for one of the inevitable lethal complications of AIDS. By then, several hemophiliac children in Colorado were diagnosed with AIDS, also acquired from blood products as had happened to Ryan White. Jonathan was intermittently quite ill and hospitalized numerous times. His lung disease persisted, and he developed another even more severe pneumonia due to a germ called *pneumocystis*. In many patients with AIDS at the time, pneumocystis was fatal. He survived it. But his survival became even more miraculous as life threw other horrific obstacles in Jonathan's path.

AIDS became one of the least of his problems.

Profiled on *Dateline NBC*, Jonathan's life story was shown to go from bad to worse. The local media covered Jonathan's AIDS infection ("Colorado's First Childhood Case"), which made him a local celebrity—and a local pariah. Like Ryan White in Indiana, Jonathan's school attendance became an intense controversy. Neighbors shunned and even threatened the family.

As the *Dateline NBC* episode detailed, churches refused entrance to the family and Jonathan was banned from the local swimming pool. The stress on the family was enormous. Tragically, the interview also revealed even more unthinkable twists and turns—Jonathan's mother's suicide attempt, her decline into crack cocaine addiction, her abandonment of Jonathan and his brother, her imprisonment for drug dealing, Jonathan's own bouts of depression. But thanks to his older brother and a saintly camp counselor, Jonathan still survived. Unimaginable.

In the mid-1990s a breakthrough in AIDS treatment occurred using a combination of three highly effective AIDS medicines at once. Jonathan inexplicably, and impossibly, survived until then and was one of the first to receive those medicines.

For me, this story came full circle today when I spoke to Jonathan on the phone. On first hearing his voice, I cried. I asked the mature adult voice on the other end if I had the right Jonathan, the one who was in our hospital in Colorado when he was just a little boy.

"Yup, that's me, man." Jonathan is thirty-two years old now and runs a restaurant in Utah with his brother, the same one who was there for him through all the earlier turmoil in his life. Jonathan was married for several years and has a child, who is now eleven years old. Neither his ex-wife nor his child became infected. Jonathan is still infected with the AIDS virus, but is healthy and the miracle of his survival continues. He continues to be compulsive about taking his AIDS medicines and about maintaining a healthy lifestyle. He is in another long-term relationship with a woman and she, too, is uninfected.

Jonathan knows how miraculous his story is—people have been telling him for years. More years than any other baby infected with this disease.

To read the complete *Dateline NBC* interview:

http://www.nbcnews.com/id/13756759/ns/dateline_nbc/t/miraculous-life-jonathan-swain/#.VcujRPlVhHw

Too Close to Home

Denise Bratcher, DO

"MIRACLES, IN THE SENSE OF PHENOMENA
WE CANNOT EXPLAIN, SURROUND US ON EVERY HAND:
LIFE ITSELF IS THE MIRACLE OF MIRACLES."

—George Bernard Shaw

As I rounded the corner to my office, I could see them already gathered in the hallway. My pediatric infectious diseases colleagues often congregate outside our offices to solicit each other's opinions when we have tough cases. One of my partners and a fellow-in-training had been consulted emergently overnight. They began to share the details of the case: a previously healthy ten-year-old boy had presented with shock and unresponsiveness and was found to have bacterial meningitis, a severe infection and inflammation of the membranes covering the brain. As I heard "ten-year-old boy," I cringed. An icy chill ran through my body as that description conjured up images of my own ten-year-old son whom I'd just dropped off at school minutes earlier.

As pediatricians, we have learned to be caring and compassionate and to treat our patients as we would want our own children to be treated, and yet one of our survival mechanisms includes maintaining enough distance to remain objective—to remain healthy. Since I became a mother, I tend to have more difficulty maintaining that separation when the children are similar in age to one of mine. This was one of those times.

It became clear, as my colleagues continued to share the details of our patient, that he was critically ill—and not likely to survive. As a result of the severe inflammation in his brain, he had developed seizure activity; he was showing abnormal posturing of his arms and legs, and one of his pupils was unresponsive to light—foreboding signs of increased swelling in his brain. In the pediatric intensive care unit (PICU), he was on a ventilator (breathing machine) and receiving aggressive treatment. The physicians involved in his care had already shared with the family that his prognosis was guarded and that he "might not make it through the night." They told his parents that he was likely to sustain brain damage as a result of this severe infection—if he survived at all—and that continued swelling in his brain could result in death. The family had called their priest, who came to the bedside to read their son his last rites.

After discussing what we could do to optimize his antibiotic therapy, we all felt the heaviness of this case as we started our day. I said a little silent prayer for our patient and turned my attention toward the rest of my day.

Later, as I walked to get my morning coffee, I ran into a family friend. As I started to ask what had brought him to the children's hospital, I instantly sensed he wasn't himself. He began to explain to me, struggling to get the words out, "It's Geoffrey. He has meningitis." Tears instantly began to stream down his face, and I felt this typically jovial, big guy crumble as we hugged. Geoffrey, his son, was the ten-year-old boy we had been talking about in the hallway earlier, and he was a friend of my son. My husband and Geoffrey's father were coaches on their youth basketball team. This amazingly athletic, smart, freckle-faced, impish boy was the kid now fighting for his life in the ICU. Any healthy distance I had established earlier was suddenly violated by the realization of this patient's identity and the need to console his father. The icy chill that I had felt initially was a harbinger of what this day would bring. I knew this kid, and I knew too much. This was too close to home.

As pediatricians, we are keenly aware that our patients are someone's son or daughter. We recognize and understand the fear that drives parental anxiety when a child is ill, and we do our best to allay those anxieties when we can while creating an honest perspective of our care. We revel in the joy and relief parents feel when their children get better and go home from the hospital. Sometimes, our patients do not survive, and every child we lose is heartbreaking. We feel the parents' loss and grieve with them while understanding that we do not walk in their shoes.

At this point, I was relieved to be able to leave Geoffrey's medical care in the capable hands of my colleagues and be his family's friend. Their church and school community held multiple prayer vigils; little prayers for Geoffrey punctuated my days and consumed my children's bedtime prayers nightly.

Geoffrey awoke from his comatose state five days later, on a Sunday morning, at exactly the time his family would typically have attended Mass— and just as his church was saying a collective prayer for him.

Remarkably, and against all odds, Geoffrey started to turn the corner, requiring less intensive support daily. He was initially left with mild paralysis of the right side of his body, which eventually resolved with aggressive physical therapy and rehabilitation efforts. Exactly three weeks after he was admitted, he walked out of the hospital to go home. The boy not likely to survive made a full recovery.

Geoffrey eventually returned to school and competitive basketball, ultimately playing varsity basketball for his high school team. During his senior year, the pediatric critical care physician who cared for him joined his family to watch one of his basketball games—a very special night for everyone. On every occasion I had to watch him play, the chills returned as I reminded my family that we were watching a miracle in action. Now, they were warm chills of gratitude. Geoffrey graduated from high school and now attends college, normal in every way.

A picture of Geoffrey leaving the hospital on discharge day still hangs outside our PICU. Every time we pass that picture, it reminds me, and everyone who cared for him, that miracles really do happen.

A Vacation Like No Other

Richard Westcott, MA, BM, BCh, DRCOG, DCH

I originally related the story of Jim in the *British Medical Journal* and revisit it now with the benefit of more than a decade of additional reflection on this case. This would be the first "miracle" in my practice, and nothing comparable has occurred since.

Jim was a submarine engineer with years of occupational exposure to asbestos. He developed *asbestosis*, a chronic lung condition from inhaling asbestos fibers. Asbestosis is characterized by lung inflammation and scarring and can result in significant breathing problems, as it did in Jim. I worked closely with Jim and his wife, Sally, a former occupational health nurse, to help get a disability pension set up for him, as his shortness of breath and weakness made further employment impossible.

As a general practitioner in the United Kingdom, I came to know Jim and Sally well over the years. I knew, for example, that Jim found his mother-in-law to be demanding and unpleasant, and I knew that Sally's back injury, which prompted her early retirement, continued to cause her pain. When Jim became diabetic, he blamed me for not making an earlier diagnosis—I countered that I tested him with the first onset of his symptoms, but we argued a bit anyway, as we were prone to do. I knew from our frequent discussions that Jim and Sally had little faith in authority, politicians, or professionals, including me it often seemed. They also had no religious faith, a position I shared with them—I am an atheist. Jim and Sally were tough characters—"hardboiled" is how I described them in the *British Medical Journal* article—yet over the years I developed a grudging affection for this couple. It's hard not to develop a personal relationship with patients in general practice when one is involved with so many serious and less serious illnesses of a couple and their family over the course of a lifetime. Jim and Sally were part of the tapestry of my career as a general practitioner.

When Jim developed a swollen right breast, he came into the office and saw one of my colleagues in the practice, who asked Jim to come back for me to check the swelling in a week or two. Jim didn't come back until many months later, when it looked for all the world as if he had breast cancer. Once more, he had cause for an argument with me about my missing something early on—that was just Jim. It frustrated us both even more when we had to repeat the biopsy several times before establishing a correct diagnosis. It turned out it wasn't breast cancer after all, but mesothelioma, a dread cancer of the linings of the lung, also associated with asbestos exposure. The tumor had spread all the way through Jim's chest wall and into his ribs and breast tissue.

We attempted radiation therapy, but to no avail. Jim became weak—and, to my great chagrin now, less argumentative. I saw Jim and Sally frequently to offer them support, but there was little else I could provide. He was deteriorating badly.

Sally decided they needed a break, and on a whim booked them on a trip to Cephalonia, an island in the Ionian Sea just west of the Greek mainland. When they returned from their holiday, they came to the office and both looked much improved! Sally asked me to examine Jim's chest—I could find no evidence of the tumor. When they saw my dumbfounded expression, they both laughed and told me this story. As I rewrite it now, I still find it all very hard to fathom.

It seems they visited a monastery on the island, of no special significance to Jim and Sally other than it was another attraction mentioned in their tour book. They were somewhat flummoxed when an old nun came up to Jim and asked him what his illness was. Sally, who wasn't sure why the nun had singled Jim out, wasn't anxious for a religious discussion or solicitation. She responded only that Jim had cancer. The nun didn't confront or engage with any of the other tourists. Shortly afterward, apparently summoned by the nun, a priest introduced himself and asked Jim to go down into a cave where a holy man used to live. Jim was too weak to negotiate the steep, narrow steps. So the priest took Jim and Sally into the church instead. The priest opened what seemed like (and, according to Sally, smelled like) a sarcophagus. Sally said they were then led through a "confused business of kissing of old rags, sprinkling of water, and mumbling," and then sometime later they found themselves outside again.

The priest again invited Jim into the cave. This time, Jim was shocked to find he could go down the steep steps and climb back up again without a problem. Since that day at the monastery, Jim has gotten stronger and healthier each day. He now stood in my clinic, astonished at his own recovery. I was speechless, but Sally pressed me for my thoughts. As I wrote in the BMJ article, "I took refuge in my role as a clinical scientist, talking about things like the body's remarkable and unpredictable powers, spontaneous remission, the delayed effects of therapy, and the benefits of a well-timed holiday." Truth be told, to this day, I still don't know what to make of Jim's recovery. Perhaps he would someday relapse, but isn't the experience of this extraordinary remission miraculous in and of itself? Isn't whatever time they gained by this remission a true gift?

I asked the couple for their thoughts. Sally wanted to scoff it off as a freak coincidence, but could not quite bring herself to deny the undeniable: her husband was recovering, and dramatically so. Each day better than the one before. Jim could only say he was "gobsmacked," or utterly astounded by this unlikely turn of events.

And so it was that one day a couple without religious faith visited a monastery. Now they and their atheist doctor had to face the question: If not this, what *is* a miracle?

To read the *British Medical Journal* article where I first described this patient, see: BMJ. 2002 Sep 7; 325(7363): 553.

EDITOR'S NOTE: Many thanks to my resourceful editor at HCI books, Christine Belleris, who tracked down the holy man referenced in this story. He was Saint Gerasimus, "the New Ascetic of Cephalonia." During the sixteenth century, after studying and serving the Church for years in Jerusalem and elsewhere in the Middle East, he was ordained a deacon and then a priest. He lived an ascetic life, with long periods of solitude. He then traveled to the island of Cephalonia, where he lived in a cave. He founded a women's monastery there, where he lived for thirty years. Legend has it that for his life of worship, servitude, and self-deprivation, he was given the miraculous gift of healing. (*http://oca.org/saints /lives/2015/10/20/103007-venerable-gerasimus-the-new-ascetic-of-cephalonia*)

DATE OF EVENT: WINTER 1979

The *Whoosh* of the Ventilator

Mary Anne Jackson, MD

As a second-year pediatrics resident on call in the neonatal intensive care unit (NICU) at night, I was accustomed to the rhythmic "whooshing" sound of ventilators (breathing machines) amid the quiet efficiency of nurses caring for newborn babies, many of whom were born way too soon and some weighing no more than a stick of butter. During the Christmas season some thirty years ago, I met "Baby G." She was not a premature baby, but a full-term newborn whose heart had failed shortly after birth. Her disease, then called *persistent fetal circulation*, caused excessive pressures in the blood vessels of the lungs, resulting in inadequate oxygen in the blood. Baby G required breathing tubes, intravenous catheters (tubes) placed in her umbilical cord for fluids, and potent medicines to maintain her heart, lung, and brain functions. The *whoosh* of the ventilator in her case was fast and frenetic, and I knew from taking care of others with her condition that her prognosis was guarded at best.

Through the night, Baby G's condition worsened and required additional support—progressively more oxygen, more ventilator assistance, more medications. Earlier in the day, air had collected in the space between her lung and the inside of her chest wall, requiring drainage tubes be placed through her outer chest wall and into her chest cavity. More tubes, more blood, more medications, but no improvement. Baby G's skin took on a purplish hue, and blood tests confirmed she was progressively worsening, the oxygen levels in her blood plummeting. We replaced her breathing tube in case the one she had was blocked, but nothing we tried worked.

At 3 AM we called Baby G's young parents, who had left the hospital briefly, and asked them to come back to the NICU because we did not think their daughter would make it through the night. They returned quickly and sat as close to their baby as they could. They held her hand and asked me if there wasn't something more that could be done. I told them we had done everything we could; I was at a loss to comfort them. Amid the ventilator whooshing, her father aloud asked God to help their baby. Her mother cried silent tears.

Baby G was in an elevated bed to allow for her care, but I wanted her mother to be able to hold her, something that had not been possible because of the baby's precarious condition. If not now, though, when? We carefully moved the baby and positioned her in her mother's arms. All fell silent in the NICU that night, except for the ventilator whoosh, until one of the nurses started saying the Lord's Prayer aloud, and other nurses followed. I stayed close by the baby as her vital signs slowly grew weaker and slower, anticipating the inevitable.

Then something happened that to this day I can't explain.

It looked as if Baby G went from purplish to perhaps less so. It was very subtle at first. Thinking it was my imagination, I withdrew a little blood from the tube in her umbilical cord artery and the previously dark blood somehow looked brighter, pinker. Now the whoosh of the ventilator seemed to blend with the prayers, harmonizing. Again I checked the blood and again it looked pinker and so did the baby's skin color. Over the next four hours, the pressures in her lungs eased and her heart and circulation continued to improve. Her parents were convinced it was a Christmas gift from God. I could not offer a medical explanation.

Still, I feared the worst was not over for Baby G. Over the previous many hours, her blood oxygen had fallen so low, and her blood acid had risen so high, as to be not compatible with life. Even if she defied all odds and survived, as it now appeared she might, she certainly would suffer severe brain damage.

At the end of the week, I went on to my next residency training assignment and did not expect to meet this little girl again. A year and a half later, though, I was working an emergency room shift, now a third-year resident-in-training. I had stepped out to the waiting room and was kneeling next to a patient's family to give them their discharge instructions. I felt a tap on my shoulder and I turned around.

"You probably don't remember me," said the father, "but you took care of my baby." I immediately recognized Baby G's father.

"There she is!" he said. "She wears glasses, but she is perfect in every way. We always wanted to tell you 'thank you' and I thought you'd like to meet her."

I turned to see a perfectly developed, adorable toddler. I get chills every time I remember our reunion. Looking at this beautiful little girl, no one would ever suspect how she started out in life, and I am still hard-pressed to explain what happened that night in the NICU.

DATE OF EVENT: 2005

A Silent Miracle

Christopher Stille, MD, MPH

It's been said that cancer in children is uncommon enough that a primary care pediatrician will diagnose only a handful of children with cancer over the course of his or her career. At the time I met Ariana, I considered myself lucky to still not have encountered my first case of cancer after almost a dozen years in practice. She was eight years old and healthy, the youngest child of three in a relatively new immigrant family from El Salvador. The family had few ties in the central New England city where we all lived, but they were a close-knit family and supported each other well. Both parents typically came to all their kids' appointments, and though neither parent was fluent in English, they learned fast. They adapted to life in this country better than most families I've worked with, helping one another in matters of language and the day-to-day struggles of running a family. After a year, their motivation, cohesiveness, and attentiveness to their health made them one of my favorite families to work with.

I saw Ariana one Tuesday morning for her regular checkup; her parents had few concerns other than she did not eat as well as their other children. She was progressing in school, making friends, and adjusting well. Her growth and development were normal, though in retrospect her weight gain over the past year was not quite as much as is typical for other kids her age. As with the thousands of other patients I had seen over the years for "well-child" visits, I started at the top for her physical exam: head, eyes, ears, nose, throat, and so on, making jokes and trying to put her at ease. I checked her neck and listened to her lungs and her heart. All normal. By the time I got to her belly, I knew I was almost done, and I began thinking about what else I needed to do to finish up this routine visit. But the next few minutes proved that this visit, this day, and the days to come would be anything but routine for this little girl, her family, and for me. To my great dismay, I felt a large, hard mass in Ariana's mid-upper abdomen.

Immediately, I had stomach pain of my own: I was certain that this was the first case of cancer in my career. *Oh no, not her*, I thought. Not believing what I felt, and not wanting to believe it, I began her abdominal exam again. I remember even shaking my right hand to make sure my fingers were working right. I felt the same thing. A huge, rock-hard mass. I completed her abdominal exam, ruling out that this was her spleen or liver in the wrong place, or stool in a constipated intestine, or a figment of my imagination. Finding the right words to communicate to the family in Spanish that I was not sure what I was feeling, but that it was not normal, became my next challenge. I asked my colleague in the next exam room to feel Ariana's belly to confirm (or hopefully refute) what I was feeling, then got a Spanish interpreter to help us, trying not to alarm the family in the process. Yet the alarm was evident in their faces.

In the next few minutes, we did our best to explain our findings and concerns to the family, and then sent Ariana for an X-ray. It confirmed that she had a mass in her abdomen the size of a small football that seemed to originate from all the way back in her spine. This was an important and potentially dire finding—large tumors emanating from the spinal cord are usually *neuroblastomas*, a potentially vicious cancer in children. The rest of my day was spent with the family in the radiology suite doing more studies and then in the oncology (cancer) clinic. We needed to quickly map out a plan to figure out how to best care for Ariana, this seemingly healthy third-grader with the small appetite.

Ariana's parents were incredible. With a couple phone calls, they calmly arranged to have their other children taken care of. They never lost their composure, despite the increasing sense of dread. They mentioned their faith in God several times, which brought tears to my eyes as I nodded and made a mental note to try to follow their example if I ever had to face something similar with my own family.

According to the American Cancer Society, there are only about 700 new cases of neuroblastoma each year in the United States. Most cases are diagnosed between one and two years of age, and 90 percent of them are diagnosed by age five years. Two-thirds of neuroblastomas have already spread to lymph nodes or other parts of the body by the time the cancer is diagnosed. Ariana, at eight years old, was going to be an unusual case no matter how it turned out, but we couldn't have imagined just how unusual.

Over the next week, we provided as much support for Ariana and her family as we could. Scans were done, surgeons were consulted, and finally Ariana had a very delicate and high-risk surgery by some of the best neurosurgeons and general surgeons with whom I have ever worked. The family and the entire treatment team felt as if we were standing at the edge of a dark and potentially dangerous forest, with some idea of the risks we faced but no certainty about how things would turn out. This tumor had to be carefully dissected away from her spinal cord by the neurosurgeons and then separated from her abdominal organs and tissues by the general surgeons. Ariana was in the intensive care unit for a few days following surgery, and she was able to go home about a week later. Fortunately, she sailed through the surgery and recovery. What could have been serious neurologic and other complications of the surgery failed to materialize.

Far more astounding was what the tumor showed when examined in the laboratory. After hundreds of microscopic sections were examined by the expert cancer pathologists, not a single malignant cell was found. I should say, not a single malignant cell *remained*, because this, indeed, had been a malignant neuroblastoma at some point during Ariana's early childhood. It had apparently completely "matured" into a benign, if enormous, *ganglioneuroma* with no effects other than that small appetite due to pressure on her digestive tract. While malignant neuroblastomas do sometimes mature into benign ganglioneuromas, tumors this large are rarely found entirely free of malignancy and without any of the complications so often seen with this cancer.

A year after surgery, Ariana had two very large scars on her trunk and abdomen, and one tiny area of decreased sensation on the front of her thigh resulting from the neurosurgeons having to dissect the tumor from the nerve root in her spinal cord where it had originated. She had no recurrence of tumor, no need for further surgery, and no need for other common treatments such as chemotherapy and radiation. And she had her appetite back!

To the family, as to me, this was a true *silent* miracle—a large and potentially terrible cancer that went away without anyone knowing it had even been there in the first place. Cancer spontaneously cured, leaving only a benign remnant as witness. And leaving a very grateful child, family, and physician.

Gracias a Dios, muchisimas gracias.

When "Alternative" Becomes the Only Alternative

David M. Polaner, MD

For an anesthesiologist and intensive care physician, life and death situations are part of the territory. We see patients every day for whom critical decisions must be made and difficult choices must be weighed, often based on incomplete or even conflicting data. We rely on our scientific knowledge and our past experience to form the best strategies, but sometimes intuition or events that seem to defy our explanations play a role, too. And, of course, when our patient is a child the consequences and emotions are magnified.

Years ago I was the director of pediatric critical care at a major New England children's hospital. We had a small staff of attending (supervising) physicians, and we were perpetually overworked. Three of us took turns covering a week at a time, twenty-four hours a day, assisted by a very talented nursing staff and highly able but relatively inexperienced interns and residents (physicians-in-training). On a Monday morning I was taking over as the attending physician for the week and making rounds with my colleague, who had just finished her very busy week as the attending physician.

We began our rounds at the bedside of the sickest patient in the unit, a little girl about two years of age with acute respiratory failure. She had been admitted a week earlier, her clinical status had deteriorated quite rapidly, and she was now receiving what might be considered maximal support with a breathing tube down her windpipe and on a ventilator (breathing machine). She had little response to our treatments and began showing signs of failure of her other organ systems. A day earlier she had been switched to a high frequency "oscillator"—a special kind of ventilator reserved for the patients with the sickest, most damaged lungs—but things had not gotten better. Despite this very aggressive management, we were making no headway improving her very low oxygen levels or reducing her sky-high carbon dioxide levels, either of which could be lethal. Increasing our sense of dread, there were new biochemical signs in her blood tests that her critical organs were beginning to show the dire effects of inadequate oxygen delivery.

Of even greater concern, this was not this child's first visit to our intensive care unit (ICU). About nine months earlier she had also been admitted with respiratory failure and barely recovered. Despite an extensive evaluation by numerous subspecialists, no cause had been discovered. Now she was back and even sicker than before, but again with no underlying cause that we could discern.

"I've begun to have discussions with her mother about withdrawing support," my colleague told me. "We are beginning to lose her, and no one can figure out what the problem is. All we are doing is providing support to keep her alive, but we're giving her no treatment of the underlying disease, whatever that is."

I understood my colleague's thinking, but something about this situation made me uneasy with the idea that it was time to give up and withdraw her support. I wasn't yet sure what I would do differently during my week on call, but it just seemed that we were not yet at the end of the line.

Our hospital was located on the edge of Chinatown, and many of our patients were recent immigrants from the Far East. This girl's family was one of them. Her mother spoke barely any English, and we relied on interpreters for virtually all communication. After completing rounds with the interns and residents, I called an interpreter and sat with the girl's mother to tell her what I thought we might change medically, to reiterate the gravity of the situation, and most of all to hear her thoughts. Speaking to parents through an interpreter is always difficult—all of the nuances that can be appreciated by face-to-face communication become diluted and difficult to discern. The cultural barriers become magnified, too. The mother listened attentively to everything I told her and replied, "I appreciate all that you are doing, but I would like to have a Chinese healer come in to help treat my daughter."

Admittedly, I am not exactly a believer in what has come to be termed "alternative medicine," but our scientific, "evidence-based" medicine had not been a rousing success either. To be honest, I was somewhat skeptical that this little girl had much of a chance of survival anyway, no matter what the treatment philosophy. We were stuck, having tried everything in our armamentarium, and despite our best efforts she was deteriorating before our eyes. It took little insight to realize that this mother needed to know that she had tried everything possible for her daughter, and that a crucial part of the formula for her included intervention by a Chinese healer.

I told her mother that we could administer the Chinese remedies only if they could be dissolved in a solution to pass through the child's feeding tube that went directly into her stomach (because of the breathing tube in her throat, she hadn't been getting food or water by mouth for many days), and only if the healer could tell us all of the ingredients. I was very concerned, because many of the ingredients in "traditional" medicines can have numerous different effects on the body, and some of those could be dangerous to a patient already in such a precarious state. Additionally, the healer's medicines could interact with drugs we were administering and cause harm. I had no objection to trying to allow the mother to feel she had done all that was possible, but I did not want the healer—and my assent to his involvement—to be the direct instrument of this girl's demise.

The next morning her condition was unchanged. The healer arrived and met with our ICU pharmacist and, through an interpreter, went over all of the ingredients. But despite extensive searching and consultation, we couldn't figure out the chemical identity of the majority of them. We decided, with much trepidation, to go ahead anyway, moved by our desire to give this mother the sense of having tried everything to save her daughter, even if her efforts were in vain.

The healer said prayers for the little girl and the Chinese medicines were flushed into the feeding tube. The rest of the day and evening passed without much change. Her oxygen and carbon dioxide levels were relatively stable with the ventilator strategy I had implemented, but her situation was still tenuous and she still required maximal support, both from our drugs and the ventilator.

By the next morning, however, we couldn't believe what was happening. She began to rally, and we were able to drop the level of breathing support we were giving her by machine for the first time in more than a week. The herbalist arrived again, and under our supervision administered a second dose of his Chinese medicines. And more prayers. By the second morning there was clear improvement, and by the end of my week on duty she had successfully weaned off the breathing machine and no longer needed the tube in her windpipe. She was now able to receive sufficient breathing support simply with an oxygen mask. The next time I came on call, two weeks later, she was no longer in the ICU at all. Several weeks after that she walked out of the hospital, fully recovered!

I learned a lot from this patient and her mother, and I think about them often, whenever I'm faced with a critically ill child. The primary lesson, of course, is that physicians should never have too much confidence in our ability to predict the future. There are surely many situations where the outcome is not hard to predict, but many where uncertainty still remains. We should never mistake one for the other, and we must have the wisdom and humility to discern between the two. The second lesson for me at this early stage in my career was to listen carefully to our patients and their families, even when you do not speak their language—both literally and figuratively.

And finally—the obvious lesson—not everything we see in our clinical practices can be explained. I will never know whether it was the passing of time, my manipulations of the ventilator settings, or the herbalist's potions and prayers that played the critical role in this girl's recovery. It doesn't really matter. In the end, all that matters is that she came back from the brink and into the arms of her family.

DATE OF EVENT: 2004

It's Alive!

Robert J. Buys, MD

I am an ophthalmologist subspecializing in diseases of the retina (the light-sensing organ lining the back of the eye) and vitreous (the fluid-filled chamber at the very back of the eye, just in front of the retina). At the time of this case, I had been in practice for twenty-one years and privileged to have participated in the care of thousands of patients both in the office and the operating room. I met incredible people, from the very young to aging World War II heroes. Of all those cases there is one that still haunts me; it can wake me up at night with a shudder. It's still the one I cannot fully explain or understand.

If you read on, it may have the same effect on you.

It all started innocently enough with a phone call. As a doctor in a referral practice, I was always happy to speak with any other physician. This one was unusual because it came from out of state and the doctor, also an ophthalmologist, seemed nervous and incredibly excited. More like talking to a kid after Christmas than hearing a calm case presentation.

With good reason. He told me that he was seeing a thirty-five-year-old healthy male who happened to work in the same building as his office. The patient was sent directly to this ophthalmologist's office when he reported to his employer he had totally lost his vision in his right eye. Examination of the eye revealed a complete blockage of the central retinal artery, causing the retina to become swollen and white. The patient's vision was barely enough for light perception, the pressure inside his eye was normal, and his eye was not inflamed. The patient reported that a similar event had occurred the night before, lasted fifteen minutes, then resolved. That history, coupled with the exam, convinced the referring doctor that a clot or a piece of calcium (called a plaque) had become dislodged and traveled through the bloodstream to the eye. He felt this "embolus" (the term for any kind of substance that shouldn't be there traveling through the bloodstream) most likely came from one of the carotid arteries, the major arteries in the neck and the source of blood supply to everything in the head, including the eyes.

That would have made sense except carotid artery clots, plaques, and emboli (plural for embolus) do not typically happen to healthy, young patients. So something was wrong with this picture, very wrong. Could this complete blockage of the central retinal artery be due to a plaque breaking off from a diseased heart valve? A normal heart exam ruled that out. Did he have some unusual disease that predisposed him to such an event? He was completely healthy and took no medications.

What was really incredible was the patient had been able to get to an ophthalmologist only minutes after the occlusion occurred because they worked in the same building. The occlusion itself is painless and can happen at any time. Once it happens, studies show you have about ninety minutes before permanent vision loss occurs. So for a patient to get proper care quickly is very rare. In all the years I practiced, the best I saw was twenty-four hours afterward. This was too late to alter the final result, which is usually vision of 20/200 or worse (considered to be legal blindness; normal vision is 20/20). That meant, for this patient, there was hope to get the presumed embolus out of the central artery and move it further downstream and preserve his eyesight. The way this is done is to lower the pressure in the eye—either by medicines, massage, or letting a small amount of fluid out of the front of the eye. With the artery facing lower pressure from the eye, it can flow more freely and hopefully push the embolus to a smaller artery, thereby creating less damage to the retina.

Then things got weird. The referring doctor said after he lowered the pressure in the eye, the embolus "emerged" from the artery, was visible for just a second, and then blood squirted into the vitreous, obscuring the view to the retina. I have never been witness to such a thing—it must have been incredible to have a front-row seat like my colleague had. What kind of clot or plaque bursts forth from a blocked artery? None that I had ever heard of!

By the time I saw the patient, about twelve hours later, my exam revealed his vision was still poor, around 20/400. There was a large clot in the vitreous which prevented me from seeing the macula, the center of vision located in the retina. But I could see the outer portions of the retina. That is when I saw what I had never seen before—and gratefully never since—a meandering, dark, narrow trail carved out beneath the retina. There is only one type of entity that can cause such a finding . . . an entity that was alive!

This was not just a piece of clot or plaque; it was a moving, living organism! Was it a parasite of some sort. A worm?

I quickly called back the referring ophthalmologist. That is when he told me the whole crazy story, one he could not believe himself. In the rush to get the patient to me and the excitement of all that had occurred, this part of the story was not originally communicated to me. He had seen some *thing* slither up from the optic nerve (where the central retinal artery emanates from). It had black and white stripes, and when it broke through the artery it looked directly at him, opening its mouth in a silent scream. He could see what looked like whiskers at the edge of the mouth, and then the blood squirted out into the vitreous obliterating his further viewing.

The phone went silent. I was shocked. I did my best to sound professional, like we see this all the time. A slithering, striped *thing* with whiskers around a gaping mouth creeping around the retina. Truth is, I was completely stunned and, between you and me, I was freaked out! *How do I treat this? Do I operate?* I'm the retinal expert after all, and I'm supposed to know what to do.

I went back to the patient and explained to him what I thought was the diagnosis. As you might imagine, that was the last thing he expected to hear from me.

We talked at great length and three potential sources of parasitic infection emerged as possible explanations: 1) he had been fishing three weeks earlier and got bitten by an insect in the eyelid; 2) he ate sushi a week before; 3) he lived in the country, near horses.

At first my concern was an infection in addition to the parasite. Clearly, this thing was from the outside world and whatever it was must have carried bacteria with it. But with no definite evidence of infection yet, I opted to wait and see what came next. Of course, I had no clue what to expect.

The next day the patient returned to my office, his eye red and with a small collection of white blood cells in the front of the eye. White blood cells are a sign of inflammation, the body's response to infection and other foreign substances. A tough call to be sure, but upon close examination I came to the conclusion the parasite had died and created an inflammatory response. The vitreous fluid in the back of the eye did not seem to have any white cells in it so I opted for conservative treatment and simply injected an antibiotic and steroid below the eye. No surgery for now.

Slowly, steadily he improved. Eventually he regained 20/40 vision. Only the remaining track of the parasite through the macula caused some visual loss. Many questions remain as I think of this: Where and how did this thing get into his body and eventually to the eye? Was there more than one? Perhaps the trail I saw was from a second parasite, the one that caused the first set of symptoms the day before he saw the referring ophthalmologist? Was there a collection of these creatures hidden somewhere else in the body? Was there a shower of these wormy creepers circulating around his body that only became apparent when one got trapped in the small retinal artery? If it had not happened the way it did, would he have ever known he was infested with parasites?

After consulting a parasite expert I concluded the most likely culprit was that a "botfly" bit him, depositing a fertile egg. Over the next two to four days, an embryo would have emerged, the textbook pictures of which match what my referring ophthalmologist had seen. From there the embryo(s) must have entered the bloodstream. But the patient gave no history of a bite in that time frame; recall the one he reported was several weeks earlier.

This is the only time I have ever seen a complete central retinal artery occlusion treated and end up with a great visual result (all credited to the rapid treatment by the referring physician who lowered the pressure in the eye and allowed the creepy crawler to move along the artery and burst through it). These occlusions almost always result in blindness. Miraculous, right? If the ophthalmologist had not lowered the pressure in the eye just in the nick of time for the little wormy parasite—striped and with whiskers around its gaping mouth—to burst forth, there would surely have been more permanent retinal damage.

Without a doubt, the most haunting, eerie, and weird case I ever treated.

EDITOR'S NOTE: To see disturbing pictures of botfly embryos (imagine these in your eye!), see: http://www.wired.com/2013/10/absurd-creature-of-the-week-botfly/

DATE OF EVENT: DECEMBER 1982

The Short Discharge Summary

Joann N. Bodurtha, MD, MPH

Following my pediatrics residency at a large, medically sophisticated East Coast children's hospital, I joined the Indian Health Service and moved to a very cold and geographically isolated Native American reservation. Overnight I went from having the best medical services in the country available to me to become a "rural medical doctor," a minimum 500-mile drive from the nearest high-level care center. My basic pediatrician's desire never to miss a diagnosis followed me, but my ability to rely on technology had changed. At night, if a patient needed an urgent blood test, I had to call a janitor to come in to drive the sample to a hospital in the next town as our testing machines weren't staffed at night. Equipment we take for granted today, like finger clip meters to measure blood levels of oxygen, wasn't available in rural hospitals.

I had previously seen this eighteen-month-old boy once in clinic. He had "failure to thrive," a condition in which growth and body weight are far below normal. This toddler was below the third percentile in weight—meaning, on a weight-for-age-and-gender growth chart, he weighed less than 97 percent of similarly aged boys—and not much interest in eating. On the very stormy night his mother brought him into our small ER, he was limp and listless, showing signs of total body failure from lack of fluids and nutrition. I knew he needed an intravenous (IV) infusion of sugar and minerals, but starting an IV line in a child this shriveled is very difficult. I tried three times, stepped away to drink a cola and regain my bearings, and tried the IV again. No luck. I was sure he was going to die, and I knew his only chance was leaving our small reservation hospital and getting somewhere where a team could start an IV surgically and provide intensive care.

I called the children's hospital in the next state, but the storm was too severe for a small medical transport plane to come. I needed to find a nurse and get our ambulance driver prepared for the twelve-hour drive with potential stops for stabilization along the way. His mother came over and held my hand several times as she saw me desperately making phone calls from our small emergency room. Our lab technician came in to help me run tests, from which I confirmed what I had already concluded from the child's deathly appearance: his blood was life-threateningly acidic. I suspected an inherited metabolic condition (a chemical imbalance caused by a genetic defect) and called the priest. The child's mother understood that he could die but wanted to try the drive, so we packed her in the ambulance with her son, the nurse, and the driver, with a map of small hospitals where they could stop along the way if he needed a final safe place.

As the ambulance pulled away, I looked up in the sky and no stars were visible through the clouds. The little boy could not possibly survive, and I knew to expect the phone call from some hospital somewhere along the way that he had died.

No call came that night, and two days later the nurse arrived back with the ambulance driver. The child's mother was staying with him in the big city. I braced myself, assuming I would hear through the reservation grapevine when he died. This would be my first pediatric death since I had arrived on the reservation. My sense of destiny and anguish about his death overrode my deep curiosity about his diagnosis and what had happened. We had no cell phones or Internet back then to facilitate communication.

It wasn't until I received the short hospital discharge summary in the mail three weeks after that starless night that I learned of the miracle. The discharge diagnosis was listed as *methylmalonic acidemia* (MMA). MMA is an inherited metabolic disorder that can be successfully managed through life with medicines and diet—but only if the patient can survive the initial crisis. Indeed, many patients don't survive the initial crisis because their deterioration has gone too far and efforts to resuscitate them are too late. This child's desperate condition that night, coupled with the prolonged delay in reaching a facility with adequate resources, put him well beyond what seemed a survivable crisis.

Yet, as impossible as it seemed to all of us involved, the brief discharge summary went on to read: "Condition on Hospital Discharge: Good."

There should have at least been an exclamation point!

DATE OF EVENT: DECEMBER 1990

A Limp Dish Rag

Adrienne Weiss-Harrison, MD

One aspect of doctoring that is rarely discussed, and about which little is written, is the "worry factor" for physicians caring for a sick patient. In pediatrics, in particular, although we must be candid and forthright with parents regarding their children's conditions, we often mask the extent of our own worry, especially if we are worriers by nature. I fall into this category, so I am conscious about trying not to let my level of concern increase parents' anxiety over their sick child. Physicians carry this "burden of worry" internally, and it is intensified by our training, which steers us toward considering the worst possible scenario when evaluating our patients and deciding upon a course of action.

It was December 1990, and a teenage patient was on my schedule one afternoon. The simple complaint on her office chart was "fever," which didn't at all prepare me for the situation that confronted me when I entered the exam room. This adolescent female appeared acutely ill with a fever over 104 degrees Fahrenheit, an extremely high body temperature for a child this age.

Based on the history given to me by the mother, my physical examination, and an X-ray, I made the diagnosis of pneumonia. To quote a phrase doctors sometimes use for the sickest kids, this young lady looked like "a limp dish rag." Many worst-case scenarios entered my mind, and I considered admitting her to the hospital directly from my office. But, since I knew the family was reliable and would return immediately if the child was not improving at home, I elected instead to give her a dose of a strong antibiotic IV (intravenously, directly into a vein) in the office, the same antibiotic she would have received in the hospital. I gave the girl's mom specific instructions about hydration, fever management, and what developments would require contacting the on-call physician and/or an emergency room (ER) visit that night. We scheduled her to come in the next day for follow-up, or sooner as needed.

As poor luck would have it, I had an appointment in New York City that evening and had to leave my suburban office right after inserting the IV line, but before the antibiotic was started. This was well before we all had cell phones to easily check in with our patients wherever we or they went.

My colleague who was on call for our practice that evening assured me he would be on top of the situation. So, I "signed my patient out" to him and drove the thirty-plus miles into lower Manhattan, thinking and worrying about this patient the whole way, reviewing the worst (and I hoped highly unlikely) outcomes, and second-guessing myself for letting this child out of my sight. The rest of the night was a blur for me. Was my patient able to take adequate fluids? Were her parents able to keep the fever down? Did she develop other symptoms? Would she need to access care in the hospital ER during the evening or night? Let's just say it was not an evening I would want to relive.

The next morning in the office, I immediately checked in with my colleague who had been on call; he had not heard from this family. I hoped for the best as I prepared to call the child's home. Just then, the nurse who had worked with me and administered the antibiotic the previous afternoon dashed in and exclaimed, "Dr. Weiss, you will not believe this! As the antibiotic was infusing, that teenage girl you saw came to life, perked up, and felt and looked much better!"

"Kathy, that's impossible," I said. "It takes an antibiotic at least twenty-four to forty-eight hours to bring a serious infection under control."

She nodded and said, "I know, but that's what happened. Really!"

The patient and her mom came in to the office that afternoon for our scheduled recheck and the next dose of antibiotic. As soon as I entered the exam room, the mother blurted out, "Wow, Dr. Weiss, that medication you gave my daughter was powerful and amazing! Before all of it even went into her arm, she improved almost 100 percent. She came back to life!"

I checked the young lady. She looked like she was ready to go out dancing, a total turnaround from the limp and listless, ill-looking teen who had been in my office just a day earlier. She was animated, dressed nicely, wore makeup, and said she felt much better. I was incredulous. Her chest sounded much clearer, too.

I told the girl's mom and our nurse that had I not seen the girl with my own eyes yesterday and then again today, I would not have believed that degree of improvement was possible in twenty-four hours, much less within moments of receiving the first drops of antibiotic. I had no scientific basis for explaining what happened.

To this day, I think about that case, and truth be told, I still cannot account for how a patient's serious infection responded so instantaneously to treatment. I was pleased that I had not shared the extent of my worry with the girl's mom, but because I hadn't, she'll probably never know that I believe a small miracle occurred that night. I learned two important lessons from this patient and what happened on those two days. Firstly, although we do sometimes face crises with our patients, thankfully, most of the time our worries about worst-case scenarios don't play out. Maybe if the worry keeps us diligent in our efforts, it's worth the toll it takes on us. And, secondly, not everything in medicine (or in life) can be explained on a logical or scientific basis.

DATE OF EVENT: SUMMER 2000

Whatever the Outcome, It Will Be Okay

David Kimberlin, MD

At the time, Casey was four years old and just starting chemotherapy for leukemia. One of the unavoidable complications of the disease and its therapy is suppression of the body's immune system, which can result in unusual and severe infections. When Casey developed eye pain and redness, along with some changes in her neurological examination, we did X-rays that showed completely congested sinuses and damage to the sinus bones. Fearing a severe sinus infection, we sent Casey for surgery to clean out her sinuses and test the contents to determine the nature of the infection.

What we found was our worst fear—a fungus infection called *Absidia*, which is uniquely seen in patients with suppressed immunity. Absidia burrows deeply into the tissues it infects, and it is almost never treatable unless the immunosuppression can be rapidly reversed—and you can't reverse the immunosuppression caused by chemotherapy on a dime the way you can with treatments for other diseases without risking worsening of the cancer. Despite the "clean-out" surgery, the fungus continued to extend into her eye socket and then her brain. Because of its location and the way it wrapped around blood vessels, we were not able to do any additional surgeries to help get the infection under control. All we were left with was antifungal medicines that usually have very harsh side effects, and we used every medical resource available to us. We even doubled the maximum dosage recommended for the antifungal medicines because her cancer was at a stage where we couldn't risk stopping her chemotherapy and we knew her immunity would continue to be suppressed for a long time. When the scans continued to show progression of the fungus deeper into her brain, with obvious destruction of brain tissue, we truly believed this was a disease she could not possibly survive. Yet she did, and to this day there is not a viable medical explanation for that miracle.

Casey lost vision in an eye and the fungus burrowed over seven inches back into her brain. Given the extent of the damage, she should have died or at the very least been severely brain-damaged. Instead we watched her course with amazement and awe. Each time I saw her in follow-up I was moved to tears because of the remarkable recovery she was making. She not only survived, but grew into a bright, interactive young woman. Her leukemia went into remission, her immune system recovered, and her fungus disappeared. *Disappeared!*

I always saw this as God's hand at work here on Earth, both in healing Casey and in guiding the family and the medical team, including me. This case occurred just after I had passed through a very difficult time in my personal life. Watching the family cope with Casey's illness was an epiphany for me, helping to strengthen my own developing faith and to teach me how to discuss God with families in the midst of crisis. Casey's parents were Christians with strong convictions; they prayed openly and frequently in Casey's room. That was not what moved me the most, though. Instead, it was the family's deep, heartfelt belief that however this turned out for their beloved daughter, it would be okay. They weren't praying for a single outcome—although, of course, Casey's recovery was their greatest hope. But, should Casey not recover, they knew, absolutely *knew*, their child would be in God's hands in heaven if not here on Earth. They were eternally optimistic that whatever the outcome, the outcome would be what God intended for their baby and for them.

I hadn't witnessed this degree of faith before, and it changed me forever. As the years have passed and I have reflected back on those miraculous events, I have learned that we usually cannot control as much as we would like to believe we can. We can, and should, do our part, but there is something bigger at work around us. Since that time, I have tried to apply my experience with Casey's parents to my professional life. I have never "preached" or imposed any belief system on the patients and families I work with, but I have become more aware of where they may be on their journey. When that includes a belief in God, I am less hesitant to acknowledge this in my conversations with them. This in turn can lead to an open discussion of faith, if the family takes the conversation in that direction. I believe that for some families this makes a true and lasting difference. Of course those families want medical treatments and cures, but they also want medical caregivers who recognize God's work in this world. I, too, benefit greatly from these deeper, more real interactions, gaining strength and wisdom from my patients and their families, and hopefully giving more of myself to them as well—not in a religious way, but in a deeper, more empathic way than ever before. My experience with my patients now is very much a shared one.

There is something bigger going on in healing than just doctors and their treatments. As caregivers, it's important to be aware that there are things out there we simply don't understand and will never fully comprehend; we must be awake and ready to listen and notice. And, sometimes, we just have to get out of the way and accept that if we've given our best effort, whatever happens will be good and right.

Casey's family never stumbled in that belief, and I have tried not to as well.

The Self-Healing Heart

Eugenia Raichlin, MD

I t had already been a busy evening when I received a call from a local hospital that was treating a twenty-three-year-old man who had suddenly collapsed at home. Michael was a second-year pharmacy student here at the University of Nebraska and had been entirely well until the past few days when he developed what he and his family thought were flu symptoms. He was desperately ill and the hospital had asked for emergency transfer to our university facility. When Michael arrived here he was pale and cold with a low blood pressure. His family was scared to death.

We did an *echocardiogram* ("echo") on his heart. An echo is an ultrasound test that allows us to see the pumping of the heart and the flow of blood through it. It's the same kind of test doctors do on pregnant women to visualize the growing fetus. The echo study shocked us: there was very impaired heart activity, minimal and ineffective contractions with minimal blood flow. The heart has four compartments, or "chambers." The lower two chambers are the ventricles, which do the pumping of blood; the right ventricle pumps blood to the lungs to receive oxygen, and the left ventricle pumps oxygen-rich blood to the rest of the body. Neither ventricle was working well—almost no blood was going to the lungs or the rest of the body.

We explained to Michael's family that we believed this was acute *myocarditis*, an inflammation of the heart muscle often caused by a virus. August was the middle of the summer flu season, and the symptoms he had earlier in the week were consistent with a virus infection that had now severely compromised his heart. No one knows why most people infected with these viruses just get a cold or "the flu," while a few develop much more serious illnesses like myocarditis. Without the heart pumping, the body cannot put oxygen in the blood or circulate the blood to the rest of the body. That explained his cold extremities and dangerously low blood pressure.

The surgeons and anesthesiologists urgently put Michael under anesthesia, put a tube into his windpipe, and connected it to a breathing machine to help him to breathe. They then connected his blood vessels to an *ECMO* machine. ECMO stands for *extra-corporeal membrane oxygenator*. This is a pump machine that circulates blood throughout the body without the use of the heart. ECMO can be used to bypass the patient's heart when it isn't functioning normally. To stay on the breathing and ECMO machines, we had to put Michael into a "medical coma," meaning he would have to be unconscious as long as he was on the artificial life support we were giving him. This was a temporary solution at best, but it was all we had. Before the ECMO machine was available, many patients with this aggressive type of heart inflammation died within hours or days.

With the family's consent, we put Michael on the heart transplant list, not knowing how long we could keep him alive on the ECMO machine. ECMO has its own potentially serious complications, including clots, stroke, infection, and bleeding. We repeated the echo imaging tests frequently to view and assess the status of his heart. What little heart function Michael had when he arrived was now almost entirely gone; blood was now stagnating in his heart! His lungs began to fill with fluid, the result of the backup of blood from his non-functioning heart. The family prayed to receive a heart for transplant before it was too late and the ECMO machine could no longer sustain Michael. Although not in front of the family, I, too, prayed to receive a donor heart to save this young man.

I was on call again over the next weekend when we received the wonderful news at night that a suitable donor heart had become available. The family was overjoyed, as were we. But by the next morning our jubilation turned to anguish—Michael had developed a fever and bacteria were growing in his blood. He had *sepsis* (sometimes called blood poisoning), a severe and potentially life-threatening infection. A heart transplant would be far too dangerous in a patient with sepsis.

Michael's family was devastated, as was I. We all believed the transplant was his last best hope. Now we were faced with a potentially tragic situation—a heart was available, but the patient was too sick to receive it. What happened next stunned us. Michael's blood pressure remained stable and even increased a bit, on its own. The heart monitors started to show signs of what looked like a slight pulse, which could not have come from the ECMO machine and therefore might reflect resumed heart activity. We hurriedly ordered another echo study and found, to our amazement, that one of Michael's ventricle chambers was now pumping. Although not yet normal, it was a dramatic improvement from the completely stagnant heart of just a couple of days ago.

We spoke with the family and advised them that we must decline the donor heart for several reasons: first, transplantation was too dangerous in the face of sepsis; second, it appeared Michael's heart was starting to "wake up"; and, finally, there was a long list of patients awaiting transplant for whom the chances of success would be greater than for Michael since the development of his sepsis. This was very difficult news for me to deliver and for the family to accept. How could we turn away a potentially lifesaving heart even if it would be a risky procedure—wasn't risky better than sure death without a transplant?

Finally, we did all agree that it was best not to put Michael through the transplant, but rather see what would happen if we gave his heart a little more time to heal itself—a concept that was not part of our thinking at all until the first signs of his ventricle contracting and pumping blood. Over the next few days his blood pressure steadily improved until we were able to take him off both the ECMO and breathing machines. His heart was now functioning well! None of us could quite believe what we had seen, but a special heart-imaging study showed only a very small and insignificant area of cardiac muscle damage in an otherwise normal heart.

If a donor heart had become available a week earlier we would have accepted it without hesitation and transplanted it into his body, removing his own severely diseased heart without giving it enough time to recover. In retrospect, that would have been a big mistake. Transplanted hearts come with great challenges—nothing is better than the organs we were born with if we can keep them working well. Ironically, his development of sepsis prevented us from making that big mistake. Now, Michael has an absolutely normal heart, his *own* heart, and didn't have to undergo the lifetime risks and challenges that go along with being a heart-transplant recipient.

Michael was the first patient at our institution to be sustained on an ECMO machine long enough to heal acute myocarditis. His experience, and that of others since from elsewhere, have now taught us to be more hopeful about the outcome in patients needing the bypass machine, and less anxious to rush to transplant no matter how dire the heart failure appears to be. This heart healed itself before we had a chance to remove it.

I was privileged to be just one of Michael's medical caregivers to witness this remarkable recovery. I am forever indebted to the fine team at the University of Nebraska who partnered in his care—his surgeons, anesthesiologists, respiratory therapists, nurses, technicians, laboratory workers, and everyone else who was committed to caring for Michael and his family. At the time, I called his recovery a miracle, and I still believe it was. Thanks to Michael and others like him since, we now have a better understanding of the potential for inflamed hearts to heal themselves. Still, the timing of Michael's sepsis event, forcing us to decline the donor heart waiting in the wings and allowing his heart just enough time to heal itself, was miraculous.

Acute myocarditis could have killed Michael. Sepsis could have killed him. He could have died from complications on the ECMO machine. Heart transplantation is risky and could have killed him. Yet, today, Michael survives with a normal heart and no long-term complications of any of his medical illnesses or interventions.

Miraculous.

DATE OF EVENT: EARLY 2000s

The Power of a Mother's Touch

Alan R. Spitzer, MD

I am a neonatologist, a specialist in the care of newborn babies. During the course of my career, I have had the opportunity to care for many premature infants born to families who struggled to conceive a child. Years ago, in the earlier days of infertility treatment, families might go through repeated courses of in vitro fertilization (IVF) in the hope of finally conceiving a successful pregnancy. This is the story of one such family and an experience that, to this day, I have no explanation for and will never forget.

In the early 2000s, the parents of Baby Daniel had several trials of IVF before finally giving birth to a tiny one-pound, five-ounce infant, delivered after only twenty-five to twenty-six weeks of gestation (forty weeks is full term). Amazingly, this baby initially did quite well, having only mild respiratory distress due to his very immature lungs. His breathing problems were fairly easy to manage with modest levels of support on a breathing machine, connected to a tube we placed through his nose and into his trachea (windpipe). A few days into hospitalization, Baby Daniel was sufficiently stable for us to initiate feedings through a tube into his stomach and begin to reduce the intravenous (into his vein) nutrition that had been sustaining the infant. The neonatal intensive care unit (NICU) staff was very pleased with the baby's progress and, in my meetings with his parents, I was cautiously optimistic about Baby Daniel's chances for survival. As always, I made sure they understood the many land mines that potentially awaited any extremely low birth weight infant during an NICU hospitalization, but I felt confident we would be able to manage this infant through those potential obstacles.

Speaking with families about their premature infants was something I always enjoyed doing, since resolving the many questions they typically had always seemed to make the NICU stay easier for everyone. If I could instill confidence in them with respect to my judgment by responding to their concerns, it added immeasurably to the ease of making the right decisions for both the baby and the parents. So each day, I would make time in the afternoon to speak with family members. I was always very keen on incorporating the family as much as possible into the care of their child; I called it "family rounds." Family rounds proved to be especially important in the events that were to follow with Baby Daniel.

Not only was this child's hospitalization one that took place in the early days of IVF, it was also early in the days of the Internet. One afternoon, when I stopped by to see Baby Daniel's parents on family rounds, they were waiting for me with a two-inch thick sheaf of articles they had downloaded online. At first, I was a bit taken aback and didn't quite know how to respond to the material they were showing me, much of which they did not fully understand. But then I realized that if I went over the articles with them and directed them to the information that seemed most rewarding, I could accomplish a few things. First, it seemed an ideal way to help educate them about the challenges facing their tiny infant and, at the same time, I could validate their desire to ensure nothing was being overlooked in the care of Baby Daniel, who was so precious to them. Furthermore, if this was to become the new approach for the parents of my future patients (and it certainly turned out to be so!), I could learn to direct their Internet searches to articles that would be most helpful to them. Baby Daniel's parents were pleased with this response, and we would typically spend ten to fifteen minutes each day going through their new downloads. Over a couple weeks, we all began to look forward to these sessions, as I found myself learning some "hot-off-the-presses" news in neonatology that I was unaware of, while the family gained confidence in my responsiveness as a physician.

Several weeks into his NICU course, however, Baby Daniel took a major unexpected turn for the worse. As was often the case, we suspected *septicemia*, a serious total body infection seen frequently in premature babies in intensive care. We obtained all the necessary tests and, while awaiting the results, started antibiotics to treat all the most common types of germs that can cause this infection. In addition, we had to increase the breathing machine support levels higher than we had ever needed for him before—an ominous sign, to be sure. Fortunately, because of our daily Internet sessions on family rounds, by this time the parents trusted my decisions and were pleased that we had reacted so quickly to the change in his condition. But over the next twenty-four hours, Baby Daniel did not respond well. His condition steadily deteriorated, forcing us to initiate a much more aggressive type of breathing support called "high frequency ventilation," along with higher and higher oxygen supplementation and increasing amounts of pressure applied from the breathing machine to get the oxygen into his stiffening lungs.

To our dismay, even these desperate measures failed to make a dent in his dangerously low oxygen levels. They continued to plummet, barely rising much above 75 percent saturation of his blood (94 percent saturation is considered normal at sea level, where we were). As a last-ditch effort to try saving his life, and years before we were fully aware of the extent of negative effects of these treatments in preterm infants, we also decided to start inhaled nitric oxide gas and intravenous steroids. I carefully explained the risks and possible benefits of these drugs to the family as best we understood them, and they were in agreement to go ahead. But within an hour, Baby Daniel's condition continued to worsen and his oxygen saturation now could barely be maintained above 70 percent, a level that will not sustain life or brain function for very long. I became quite sure that all was lost and death was imminent.

When a child's condition reached the point where I felt death was a certainty, I always believed it was important for a family to hold their infant, even if only for a brief time, so it was clear to them that however short the infant's life, it would always be real and a part of their consciousness forever. At the time, "kangaroo care" (named for the way marsupials carry their infants, and first practiced with pre-term infants in a facility in Bogota, Colombia, in the late 1970s) was a relatively new practice in American NICUs. It involves direct skin-to-skin contact between a baby and his mother. In practice, for a premature infant like Baby Daniel, the first step was to make sure the breathing tube in his throat was carefully secured with tape to his face. He would then be placed naked, except for a diaper, on his mother's chest. Although now commonly practiced in many nurseries, and especially useful for premature babies to enhance bonding, we hadn't had much experience with this technique, but I felt it would be an ideal way for this mother to hold her dying child one last time.

With the assistance of the nursing staff, we cautiously moved Daniel from his warmer bed and placed him on his mother's chest. She asked me how long he had to live, and I told her that at some point, as his oxygen levels continued to decline, we would simply discontinue the breathing machine support and make him comfortable with medication to ease any terminal discomfort he might have. It would be a gentle way to die but, needless to say, everyone in the room was profoundly saddened for this lovely family who so wanted this child. I began to go through the usual inner recriminations of what I had missed, where I had failed, what could I have done differently.

What happened next, I have no explanation for, and I do not recall another child I have ever cared for where my assessment of imminent death was so wrong. I turned to Baby Daniel's oxygen saturation monitor, expecting the value to have fallen further on its way to his death, but to my astonishment, since being placed on his mother's chest his oxygen saturation had suddenly risen to 92 percent! The baby's color, which had been gray and ashen, suddenly appeared pink and rosy. His father, seeing the puzzlement on my face, asked me what was wrong. I told him nothing was wrong and, in fact, this was Baby Daniel's best oxygen saturation level in many hours. His mother asked me what we do now, and I told her we should just wait and see, but this was likely to be just a brief interlude and they shouldn't get their hopes up too high.

As if to mock me, the oxygen saturation continued to climb over the next few minutes, rising to 95 to 96 percent. The baby went from oxygen saturation plummeting toward death to an absolutely normal oxygen level within mere moments of lying down on his mother's chest. At that point, his mother said to me that she was absolutely not moving from her chair. And she didn't for the next two days, only allowing for brief respites during which time she would allow her husband, and *only* her husband, to slip in and replace her in holding the baby. Her husband's chest was quite hairy, and during his time with the baby, it almost appeared as if the tiny infant vanished in a forest.

With this remarkable parental addition to our therapy, Baby Daniel steadily weaned from the high-frequency ventilator, went back to the conventional breathing machine, and continued to improve from there. Almost unimaginably, he was discharged home a few weeks later. I was able to follow him for several years and he did wonderfully, even winning a soap-box derby in his home town at about age eight. His proud mother sent photos of the event to me.

With all the high technology in our NICUs, and the newest innovations in the care of premature babies, Baby Daniel reinforced for me the irreplaceable impact of parental love in altering an infant's outcome, no matter how small the baby, and no matter how ill. I wish I could explain what happened that day in our NICU. But for Baby Daniel, his parents, and for me, it was very real, very powerful and, perhaps, even miraculous.

3

Breathtaking Resuscitations

When the heart stops, the clock starts. Without adequate blood and oxygen circulation to the brain and other vital body organs, permanent damage or death occurs. The longer the cardiac arrest lasts, the more likely there will be a tragic outcome.

The essays in this chapter describe patients whose hearts were stopped far longer than should be survivable, despite desperate attempts at cardiopulmonary resuscitation (CPR) by skilled and trained personnel. After being pronounced dead, or presumed to be brain dead, the miracles began.

DATE OF EVENT: MARCH 2015

A Spirit of Calm, an Aura of Awe

Frank Maffei, MD

Richard L. Lambert, MD

Gardell was the lead story in all the local, national, and international news media.[1-5] "Toddler Survives after 101 Minutes of CPR." "Pennsylvania Toddler Survives Near-Drowning after 101 Minutes of CPR." "Miracle Toddler Who Fell in Stream Brought Back to Life after 101 Minutes of CPR." "Toddler Dead for 101 Minutes Is Now Alive." "Toddler Revived after Nearly 2 Hours of CPR." But no media description could do justice to what we saw happen before our eyes that night and morning.

It was mid-March and the pediatric intensive care unit (PICU) where I work was still busy from a winter that brought us severe respiratory disease and a facility filled to near capacity. I was coming on call for the evening and had just been briefed on all the patients in the PICU from my partner and close friend, Dr. Richard Lambert, who had been on call before me. As he finished going through the youngsters' cases one-by-one, a call came from one of our emergency department (ED) physicians: "I don't have all the details yet, but there is a two-year-old boy who drowned and they have been doing CPR (cardiopulmonary resuscitation) for over forty minutes. We may decide to stop the CPR once we fully assess, but just giving you a heads-up." A mere moment after I hung up, I thought about a run I had taken by a lake just the day before, and remembered there was still ice on the surface. I called the ED back.

"Was this a bathtub drowning or was this an outside drowning?"

"It was a creek but we don't know much more," he answered.

I responded, "Do not terminate CPR; let's assume this was a true ice-water drowning."

It turns out the local Emergency Medical Service (first responders) team and community hospital where the child was first taken were assuming exactly that, and they diligently continued high-quality CPR without interruption. In an ice water immersion, hypothermia (low body temperature) is the primary event and cardiac arrest follows. In these rare cases, the initial deep hypothermia produces a state where the human body has very low metabolic and oxygen needs. This may lead to a protective effect on vital organs, in particular the brain. But there is a limit as to how long the vital organs can survive even with deep hypothermia. Had this little boy passed that limit?

As I left my office for the ED, Rich went to quickly scour the most recent scientific literature for any new and useful information pertaining to hypothermic drowning. He would then join me to assist with the child's resuscitation. When we arrived in the ED, the highest level trauma alert had been sounded and there were more than enough personnel standing by ready to help.

That being said, even with the best intentions, too many sets of hands can lead to chaos. We took the ten minutes prior to the helicopter landing to quickly assign roles and places. We had key staff ready to do the primary evaluation, airway management, heart monitor and breathing machine set-up and, of course, CPR. We assigned four doctors to line up on the toddler's left side and rotate every two minutes to provide high-quality chest compressions. CPR is very tiring to perform and can quickly lead to exhaustion of the person performing it. The ED doctor who made the initial call to me earlier would oversee the CPR and keep track of time and medications being administered. Rich and I would do the initial examination, attempt to insert IV (intravenous) lines, and guide the rewarming strategies. I called our heart surgeon and asked him to be ready to place the child on a cardiopulmonary bypass machine for rewarming if our efforts in the ED did not result in a return of spontaneous circulation. Cardiopulmonary bypass is the same technique used for open-heart surgery, a pumping machine that takes over the job of a patient's heart and lungs. By warming the blood in the machine, it can also be used to rapidly warm a hypothermic patient's core body temperature.

I could hear the helicopter landing. The crew reported: "Two-year-old went missing at 6 PM for 30 minutes. EMS was dispatched. Neighbor found him a quarter mile downstream in a swollen icy creek that runs past the back of the yard. CPR was started a minute or so after he was pulled from the creek and has been continuous since. Accounting for the scene, the stop at the community hospital and the helicopter flight here, we have CPR for one hour and 16 minutes. Gardell's initial rectal temperature was 25 degrees Celsius (77 degrees Fahrenheit)." So that was 30 minutes of the child being missing and 76 minutes of CPR with a core body temperature more than 20 degrees below normal. Surely this was pushing the limit of even the most dramatic ice-water drownings.

The resuscitation was transitioned from the transport crew to us, and immediately we were all struck by the spirit of calm in the room. Everyone had a role, everyone knew how to perform that role, and we all had a shared purpose: save this little boy if at all possible. We didn't dare allow ourselves at that moment to think it might not be possible. Some of those doubts started a little later.

Start at the top. The child's airway was secured with a tube in his trachea (windpipe), allowing the ventilator (breathing machine) to breathe for him. We determined our CPR heart compressions were effective and we could hear appropriate air movement in his lungs from the breathing machine. Yet, Gardell had absolutely no signs of life. No movement, no response of his pupils to light, no response to pain, no breathing on his own, no heart rate. He looked awful, worse than awful, but something told me he was still in there, that he was not truly dead.

Get to work. The ED doctor kept track of the CPR, vital sign monitors were activated, and then we needed to get him warm. Cold would no longer be protective at this point, and in fact prolonged cold could now do more harm than good in our efforts to revive this little boy. Warming blankets were placed around him and warmed, humidified oxygen was delivered through the tube in his trachea. Warm fluids were flushed in and out of his stomach and urinary bladder. This all occurred within minutes of his arrival amidst that spirit of calm determination from everyone in the room. I don't think I'd ever before experienced that universal calm in a situation as harrowing as this. So much was getting done, still without any sign of life; there was much more that still needed to happen.

While cold may temporarily protect the vital organs, it does so at a price—blood vessels throughout the body leading to and from the body's surface clamp down and finding veins for IVs can be very difficult. For that reason we had initially relied on a special type of IV, called an *intraosseous* line, directly into the little boy's bone marrow. "The intraosseous line is not working well," someone called out. We needed access to a large main vein immediately.

I looked at Rich, "I'll go to the neck and you go to the groin." It's tough enough to get an IV into a major blood vessel in small children, but in a youngster who is cold and being bounced around from the CPR, it can be nearly impossible. We knew we would have to temporarily stop the CPR to get access into a large central vein, but also knew we had to minimize any CPR interruptions, so we timed our needle punctures together.

"Ready . . . stop CPR, now." Almost immediately, and almost too easily, we both succeeded in putting IV tubes in the large veins of the neck and groin, allowing us to give Gardell warmed IV fluids and medications as close to the heart as possible. His temperature was now up to 84 degrees Fahrenheit but still no signs of life. Emergency medicines intended to jump-start his heart and treat the acid that builds up in a body under these circumstances were repeatedly given but with no change in his status.

"Is the heart surgeon getting an operating room (OR) ready for the bypass machine?" I asked.

"Yes, it'll be ready in five minutes."

Now, as we contemplated escalating the resuscitation to the bypass machine, doubts began to surface among some of our colleagues.

"Dr Maffei, how long will you go here? It's been an hour and thirty minutes. At what pH would you consider stopping?" The pH refers to the amount of acid in the bloodstream—the longer a patient's tissues are deprived of oxygen, the more acidic the body becomes. And the more acidic the body becomes, the less likely it is that vital organs, especially the brain, will ever recover. In my entire career, I've never cared for a child that survived with a pH less than 6.5, and surviving doesn't necessarily mean surviving with an intact brain.

"We don't stop until he is rewarmed to 90 degrees Fahrenheit, and I don't really know about a specific pH but if you want a number, anything less than 6.5 is likely to be non-survivable."

"His blood gas results are back," someone called out. I held my breath while the numbers were read aloud. The blood oxygen was far too low, the blood acid level was far too high, and "The pH is 6.504."

Now what? I thought. While the pH of 6.504 *is* greater than 6.5, the difference is less than negligible. But the pH wasn't *less* than 6.5. I was grateful that a voice inside of me had chosen 6.5 as my make-or-break number because that same voice inside of me had told me we shouldn't give up, we still had a chance. We prepared Gardell for transfer to the OR, where he would be put on the cardiopulmonary bypass pump. The transfer from the ED to the OR went seamlessly without having to interrupt CPR. The heart surgeon and his team were scrubbed and sterile and ready to go.

I decided we would do one last pulse check and then Gardell would be in the surgeon's hands for the bypass procedure, which we all knew carried its own significant risks. No machine can mimic the effectiveness of the body's own heart and lungs, and cardiopulmonary bypass is no exception. Patients on the "pump" are at risk for stroke, bleeding, even further heart damage, kidney damage, infection, and other complications. It was a huge step to take, especially since we didn't even know if we had a chance for normal brain function after the prolonged drowning and resuscitation efforts.

"Rich, I'll check his groin artery for a pulse if you check his neck artery. Everyone, please hold on your CPR for a moment while we check for a pulse and heart rhythm."

"I have a pulse," Rich and I said confidently and simultaneously. We looked at the monitor. Normal heart rhythm at 70, then 80, then 100 beats per minute with a blood pressure of 78/44—good enough. We again held our breath waiting to see if this could be sustained; we detected no abnormal rhythms, only a stronger and stronger pulse and improved blood pressure each minute.

There would be no hooting or hollering, no slaps on the back, no high fives—only that same spirit of calm determination we had experienced from the beginning, but now with a profound sense of peace and thankfulness. Yet we all knew enough to also feel nervous trepidation of what lay ahead. A beating heart did not necessarily mean a functioning brain.

Little Gardell did not need the cardiopulmonary bypass machine, but there was still much more work to do: fine tuning his breathing machine, slow and cautious rewarming, continued careful monitoring of his core vital signs, medication adjustments, corrections of abnormal laboratory findings, and watchful waiting in the PICU defined our night. After all the stabilization and high-intensity activities, I could finally breathe long enough to begin to meet the family. First, I met with Gardell's pregnant mother and then, one by one, his six siblings. The little boy's father, a truck driver, was racing home from Detroit to be with his son. They were all tearful but hopeful. This is a deeply religious family; they pray and turn to God for all things.

I also took a moment to look at some of the scientific literature and data Rich had found earlier in the evening. Not good. Yes, rare cases of meaningful survival after ice-water drowning with prolonged resuscitation do occur, but fatalities or severe neurologic disability are far more likely the outcome. As my own professional experience had taught me, and as that inner voice had told me during the resuscitation, I couldn't find any reports of a survivor who had an initial pH of 6.5 or lower. *What have I done?* Have I saved the heart and lungs of a child only to create a vegetative state? What will Gardell's brain function be like after such an ordeal?

I finally pray, "Lord, help this child and his family—be with them. Stay with me, as I felt your presence during his resuscitation."

It was now 2 AM in the PICU. I was in the unit watching over our nearly frozen toddler and gently, quietly, speaking to his family. "We will do everything we can for Gardell. We may not know for days what the extent of his recovery will be and indeed even his survival is still in question." The family left the PICU to get some rest on the chairs and floor of our waiting room.

At 3 AM the tube in his artery that was providing blood pressure readings malfunctioned. That could have been bad news. I hoped it was just a mechanical problem that required some troubleshooting rather than requiring the replacement of another tube. I went to the bedside to check on it and I did a double-take, and then a triple-take. Was he trying to open his eyes? I called to the bedside nurse, "Did you just see that?"

"Amazing," she replied, "amazing."

A short time later, he again opened his eyes and looked straight at me. I called his name and he grimaced. "Gardell, do you want to see your mommy?" I asked.

He nodded, an unmistakable "Yes!" We called his family in immediately, including his father who has arrived just in time to witness his baby's remarkable and stunning awakening.

After only eight hours since his pulse had returned, Gardell was now answering questions. Word spread fast: every doctor, doctor-in-training, medical student, night nurse, aide, and respiratory therapist stood around his bed dumbfounded and overjoyed. As we all looked at Gardell, his family, and each other, there was again a spirit of calm and peace in the room, now with an aura of awe.

"Do you want to play trucks when we go home?" his father asked Gardell. He smiled around the tube still in his throat. I stood back and thanked God.

A day later, Gardell was liberated from the breathing machine and, a mere three days after being pulled, frozen and dead, from an icy stream, Gardell went home from the hospital. His mom sent me a beautiful video showing Gardell running and playing with a balloon his siblings gave him.

Gardell went on to make a full recovery.

I often stop to think about how we got from an hour and forty-one minutes of CPR to a happy and beautiful little boy who can bounce a balloon with his brothers and sisters. I reflect on the more than fifty people whose complete and total devotion to saving this child did, indeed, save him: the neighbor who searched far down an overflowing stream to find him facedown in the water, stuck on a branch; the incredible first responders who knew not to give up on their CPR; the dedicated physicians and nurses at two hospitals who orchestrated a phenomenal resuscitation. Calm, but determined heroes, every one of them.

Most of all however, I am left with the overwhelming sense that divine guidance enabled us to resuscitate Gardell. Many of us have since remarked that there was never a feeling of desperation or hopelessness throughout the entire resuscitation. It was as if we were hearing from above, "Do your job and I will take care of the rest."

---

1 *http://www.cnn.com/videos/tv/2015/03/20/lead-pkg-darlington-toddler-revived-after-near-drowning
.cnn*

2 *http://www.nbcphiladelphia.com/news/weird/Toddler-Survives-CPR-Pennsylvania-Icy-Creek-29695
4871.html*

3 *http://www.mirror.co.uk/news/world-news/miracle-toddler-who-fell-stream-5377435*

4 *http://fox8.com/2015/03/20/toddler-dead-for-101-minutes-is-now-alive/*

5 *http://abcnews.go.com/Health/video/pennsylvania-toddler-revived-after-having-no-pulse-for-hours
-29781706*

DATE OF EVENT: JANUARY 2009

The Miracle of Teamwork

Paul A. Skudder, MD

L ate afternoon on a Monday, I was visiting the cardiac intensive care unit (ICU) and had to introduce myself to the nursing staff; I'm not in the cardiology department and they did not know me. I asked a few questions to locate a patient who did not expect to see me.

There were several family members at his bedside, concerned but looking ever so much more relieved than when I had last seen them. Far more relieved. And the patient, in his late sixties, was smiling, sitting up, a bunch of tubes coming from various body locations, cheerful and speaking with his family. A new man, a new lease on life. *Wow.*

I began, "Do you recognize me?"

"No . . . should we?"

"Well, maybe, maybe not. It's a bit out of context," I answered.

I thought, *Like really way out of context. All they see is another doc in a white coat and a tie, in a big hospital where docs in white coats and ties are a dime a dozen. I'll bet they've seen so many docs in the past two days they couldn't recognize half of them.*

But they wouldn't remember me from the hospital. It was before all of this. Before the helicopter. Before there was hope.

They looked at me some more. I reached into my pocket, the pocket of my white coat that usually holds my stethoscope. I pulled out a baseball cap with a logo on it. I put it on slowly. I adjusted it and I smiled.

Stunned silence.

✧ ✧ ✧

Back to two days earlier. It's frigid, just a couple degrees above zero. Crystal clear, visibility from here to everywhere. A busy Saturday in the ski industry, a mountain full of enthusiastic customers enjoying a "bluebird day," the kind where the snow is fluffy and soft, the air is crisp and cold, and your skis seem to turn effortlessly. At the summit of the mountain, in the old wooden shack, those ski patrollers who are not out scanning for the injured, cold, or lost are warming up last night's leftovers in the old microwave with the broken handle. It's time for lunch, and the homemade wooden table is surrounded by familiar faces, relaxed, going over the last few days' challenges, pondering how long the weather will remain clear and cold, and wondering who was on duty next weekend. Generally just "chewing the fat" as they say. The desk is manned by the dispatcher. There are two phones, two radios, and a logbook full of scribbles nobody could really read. The dispatcher turns to me and barks over the crackle of a radio:

"Hey Doc, they are starting CPR (cardiopulmonary resuscitation) on the snow in front of the mid-mountain restaurant."

Red coat on quick, helmet buckled. Turn on my two-way radio hustling out the door. Yell something about "Somebody be sure the portable de-fib is on the way." That's the defibrillator machine we use to restart stopped hearts; you know, the "paddles." *Snap, snap* into my skis. Push hard away from the shack, over the little hump and point them *down*. Don't turn, don't brake. Just go, go, a mile and a half to go, just go. Wind whistling by, biting and cold, freezing exposed skin. Chatter on the radio. Others coming, gathering, different skills assembling. Turn hard, staying on the shortest path between two points. Around the corner, avoid the customers, don't cause another problem. Over the last hump, and there they are, the first of our highly trained team to arrive, red coats, white crosses on the back of each one, bent low, on their knees. Around him.

The group makes room for me. CPR chest compressions (pumping) underway, bare chest, defibrillation pads are already in place. It's cold, maybe four degrees Fahrenheit, his bare skin is blue, lips blue, face ashen, his whole body bouncing on the snow with each compression. A breathing mask held over his nose and mouth, attached to a bag squeezed regularly, pushing oxygen from a small green torpedo tank into his lungs.

Too many spectators; scared family, curious onlookers. "Get crowd control! We need room to work!"

"We can talk to family later."

"Everybody *clear!*"

The defibrillator fires. "Shock delivered!"

Compressions again. Shock again. No response. He needs meds, he needs meds. Medicines are crucial for resuscitation of a heart attack patient. Continue compressions. Trade off, somebody else give compressions. He is cold. Maybe that's good, they use hypothermia (low body temperature) intentionally in intensive care units after heart attacks, protects the brain and other organs. He's cold. Stay on it.

More noise, a roar, a gasoline engine, smells like an outboard. The crowd parts. Snowmobile skids in next to us. Meds have arrived with licensed personnel. Open the box, root around, find the meds we need, draw them up in a syringe, push them in the vein. What vein? They are all collapsed, it's freezing. Veins collapse in the cold. Nobody can find a vein; too cold, too constricted. Where is the biggest needle? Gotta find a really big vein. His neck, look at the neck, find the "landmarks," the jugular vein will be there even though we can't see it. "*Stop compressions!*"

"Why? No! He needs compressions!"

"Stop, I can't go for the jugular with the man bouncing like this." Without meds he'll die. Stillness. One pass, straight into the jugular. Yes, we have an IV line! Start pumping again, CPR compressions. Where are the meds? Here, here, push them in here. Epinephrine (aka adrenaline) pushed into the jugular IV. Compressions. Shock. Repeat. Epinephrine. Compressions. Shock.

Off, everybody off. Check him. He has a pulse. No? *Yes!* Cover him, get him warmed up. Maybe? Is it better if he's cold? Where is the two-passenger

CPR toboggan? Here it is—great, already here. People are thinking and moving. A team! This is why we practice so hard.

Strong guys, big guys to steer this one down the mountain! He's a big guy and we need a rescuer on the toboggan with him to squeeze the air bag that's providing oxygen for him, breathing for him. He's not conscious. Will he live? Pupils dilated, a bad sign, will he wake up? We don't know, can't say. Yes, his pulse is still there. Good. Blood pressure? Yes, he has a blood pressure. No bleeding. Cardiac event. Call air ambulance, this one needs a chopper.

He needs a breathing tube in his windpipe before we can put him on the chopper. Wow, these guys with military field experience are good; in the tube goes, on the ground, on the snow. Putting that tube in can be tough in a hospital, on a bed, with bright lights and all the rest! This is now an ICU in the snow, artificial breathing apparatus, jugular IV lines, meds, all of it!

The chopper is on the way. Skiing down, down, a careful two miles on the snow. Strong skiers pulling, two men in the toboggan, one breathing for the other, keeping him alive. Not too fast, don't lose control, don't roll them over, but no time to waste. Air ambulance arrives. Tell the flyers the story, details, what we did, how he is. Load him up, strap him in. Off he goes.

Now the family, ask them about it. Crying; fear; what happened? What will happen? Heart attack? No better explanation at hand, he just dropped on the snow after lunch in the restaurant. They say he was happy all morning, no complaints, no warning signs. Just went down after lunch. Yes, we did our best; we hope he will make it. Do you need directions, how to drive from here to the hospital, almost two hours?

Good luck. God be with you. Best to drive carefully; hurrying will not help him.

❖ ❖ ❖

Where were we? Oh yeah. I reached into my pocket, the pocket on my white coat that usually holds my stethoscope. I pulled out a baseball cap with a logo on it. I put it on slowly. I adjusted it and I smiled.

Stunned silence.

Then . . . "Are you one of *those guys*?!"

The red-and-white logo on the cap read SKI PATROL.

"Yup. One of those guys. The one with the big needle."

So the visit began, smiles, tears, hugs all around. Memories of an eventful day from different perspectives. Talk of the procedures in the hospital since then, the diagnosis of the heart attack, and the cardiologists' good care to ensure a good outcome.

"No, I was not involved in the procedures in the hospital, I am not a cardiologist. I am in a different field of medicine. I did my part the other day. I volunteer at the mountain, part of the patrol, there to help. It's a really good team."

DATE OF EVENT: 1999

A Good Samaritan Repaid

Fred M. Henretig, MD

It was a lovely spring weekend, but it was my lot to be working a Saturday shift as the attending (supervising) physician in the emergency room. The morning had begun with nothing out of the routine for our busy, urban children's hospital—lots of sick, feverish infants, children of all ages with minor trauma, children with asthma and other chronic illnesses having flare-ups—yet happily, no catastrophic events to confront so far that day. That all changed when we heard the hospital operator on the overhead paging system call "Code Blue," the emergency code for a patient having a severe, potentially life-threatening heart or breathing problem.

But, rather than the usual location announcement directing physicians, nurses, and technicians to a *patient's* room, this call was to the elevator located in the center of our lobby. That was unusual, but even more unusual for us was the patient—a middle-aged adult who was visiting the hospital that day. We don't often treat adults in our children's hospital, and I must say it made me more than a little nervous. It had been over twenty-five years since I graduated medical school and entered into pediatrics, and even though all of us in the ER had taken the standard courses in adult life support and cardiopulmonary resuscitation (CPR), this situation was definitely out of my comfort zone! Apparently this man had entered the elevator on the first floor and immediately collapsed when the door opened onto the eighth floor.

We later learned this wonderful gentleman had volunteered to donate his Saturday as a chaperone for a group of New Jersey high school students who had come to perform their class play, *The Wizard of Oz*, for our hospitalized children, providing a little good fun and distraction from their illnesses. He was accompanying his longtime partner, a lovely woman who was one of the school's math teachers and also assisting the senior class play director.

The group entered the elevator on the first floor and planned to exit on the eighth floor where they were going to entertain the patients. The elevator was very stuffy, packed with the students and chaperones. Our patient had taken a nitroglycerin tablet (for chest discomfort) before entering the elevator. When the elevator door opened on the destination floor, he fell face down in the elevator and stopped breathing. He never made it out of the elevator and someone started CPR immediately. The high school students exited the elevator, the hospital representative greeting the students used the elevator phone to contact the hospital emergency operator, and the elevator went back down to the first floor where we, the ER team, met our patient for the first time. He was in full cardiac arrest, without a discernable heartbeat. We continued CPR as we lifted him onto a gurney and wheeled him back to the ER. There, we quickly attached wires to leads taped on his chest to obtain an electrocardiogram (EKG) assessing his heart function, and placed a breathing tube into his main airway, the trachea, to provide rescue breathing.

We found him to be in *ventricular fibrillation*, the most serious of all abnormal heart rhythms. In *V-fib*, the heart muscles in the pumping chambers quiver rather than contract as they normally should, and as a result no blood is pumped to the body. We continued performing CPR, as well as giving him emergency heart medicines and using paddles to try shocking his heart back into a normal rhythm, for almost an hour. He repeatedly—at least ten times—would seem to have a return of a weak pulse, suggesting some return of a heartbeat, but it would last only a few seconds, and then quickly revert back to his life-threatening V-fib rhythm.

As the team leader of this resuscitation effort, I found myself to be in an increasingly difficult situation, despite having directed dozens of pediatric resuscitation efforts over my years in practice. Many of the nurses at the bedside had come to think that we had lost this patient, and that prolonging a "futile" effort was becoming disrespectful of the (presumably) newly deceased patient's body, as well as cruel to his partner, who was with us in the resuscitation bay the whole time all of this was going on. I was asked several times if it wasn't yet time to "call the code," meaning stop the resuscitation. But I had my doubts that it was time to let go. The recurrence of even a faint pulse, though very briefly, suggested some life was yet there in this man's heart. And perhaps my hesitation was furthered by a sense of insecurity, given my relative lack of experience with treating adult heart disease, and yet being in charge of this situation.

Fortunately, one advantage of working on a team in a teaching hospital medical center is that we always have a variety of staff participating. We had already called our affiliated adult hospital next door, describing the situation and asking if any other approaches might help; they really didn't have much more to offer. Still, I asked if one of the team there might be able to make the five-minute dash across the alleyway, and of course they offered to send someone right away. But just as we were getting closer and closer to ending the resuscitation effort, one of the bright young physicians-in-training who was already assisting us at the bedside had an idea. He was a resident in adult emergency medicine, assigned for a month to our children's hospital to become more familiar with pediatric emergencies. Before coming to us, back at his home hospital, he had recently seen the senior physicians try a new drug to treat V-fib victims who were unresponsive to the standard battery of medicines. This new medicine was *amiodarone*, a drug that was rapidly gaining usage in the adult cardiology world and, as it happened, even by pediatric heart specialists for certain special cases. It turns out our cardiologists had arranged for amiodarone to be stocked in our hospital's main pharmacy, but it was so new and reserved for such special cases that we did not even stock it in our emergency department yet! I didn't hesitate once the trainee in adult ER medicine made the suggestion—what was there to lose? We rushed a request to our pharmacy, and within minutes it was "special delivered" to us in the ER.

Remarkably, our patient had a great response to the amiodarone. Almost immediately after the infusion was completed, he returned to normal heart rhythm, with a strong pulse and nearly normal blood pressure. This time, his improvement persisted, not relapsing to V-fib. Just then, our adult emergency medicine colleague from next door arrived and arranged for urgent transport from our ER to their cardiac intensive care unit. We all breathed a deep sigh of relief and hoped for the best. I still had the sense that several of my coworkers thought we had gone on too long, that surely after more than an hour of being kept barely alive by CPR, his prospects for meaningful recovery were dismal.

Later that day those fears were only heightened. I had dispatched one of our pediatric ER trainees to visit the cardiac unit next door to find out what was happening. She reported back to me that the cardiology team had immediately performed a procedure to diagnose the condition of the man's heart's arteries and expand a small balloon within them to improve blood flow. They discovered he had several severely blocked heart arteries and intended to take our patient directly to the operating room to try to surgically "bypass" his clogged heart arteries.

Alas, as per the cardiologists' routine after a prolonged resuscitation, a comprehensive neurologic evaluation was done first, which revealed signs of massive brain injury. His partner later recalled to me that the heart surgeon arrived with another physician, introduced as the neurology specialist, who told her that "It was worse than they thought," that likely not enough blood had gotten to his brain during the nearly hour-long absence of normal heart function, and that he had suffered irreversible brain damage. The neurologist cautioned her that the probability of his ever awakening was next to nil, and the heart surgeon had therefore decided he was no longer a surgical candidate.

I went home that evening with very mixed emotions. I had for a brief few hours believed we may have saved a man's life, and I was proud of being "stubborn" about my instincts and refusing to quit the resuscitation. But now I was left to wonder if my decision, and all our efforts, had only resulted in a man having to "live" on a breathing machine, in a vegetative state. It did occur to me that during his resuscitation we had used multiple doses of powerful drugs for his abnormal heart rhythm, which often have a deeply sedating effect. I wondered if that might have impacted his later neurologic exam, yet still wear off eventually. But surely the neurologists had taken that into account.

And yet, despite this grim turn of events, the story of our Good Samaritan volunteer had a happy ending. His partner never lost hope, despite the grim prognosis. She and other friends and family members kept a vigil at our patient's bedside and applied several alternative medicine healing techniques to him that they felt comfortable with. He did require considerable traditional medical support for the first day or two, with multiple medications for his heart and blood pressure, as well as sedatives to keep him from "fighting against" the breathing machine that was keeping him alive. His heart function improved dramatically, and after being kept in deep sedation for several days, the cardiac care team let his sedating medications wear off, to see what would happen. Was there any brain function left?

To everyone's amazement, he rapidly woke up! Soon, his doctors were able to take him off the breathing machine entirely. To this day, I have a picture on my desk of him sitting up in bed just four or five days after the ER encounter, with his loving lady by his side, her arms around him. They were home within two weeks. Six months later he thoughtfully came back to look me up and say thanks to all of us. We visited the resuscitation room in our ER, met the nurses who'd been there that day, and then I took him back to the adult hospital next door to revisit that site.

We spent most of that afternoon together, and I had a strong impression that this man was intellectually 100 percent intact. He had a charming sense of humor, cautious optimism about his life to be, and a sense of wonder and gratitude for having survived. It also gave me the chance to tell him it wasn't really me who saved his life. Rather, it was a cluster of small miracles, serendipitously aligning just in the nick of time. He suffered his deadly abnormal heart rhythm while in a hospital where there were many skilled health professionals only a few feet away. One of those skilled people, still in his training and on a most fortuitously timed tour of duty with us, happened to have used a new medicine none of us had experience with. That medicine was available right in our own hospital (if not quite yet in the ER) and accomplished what none of our efforts up to that point had been able to accomplish. In the years since, amiodarone has become a staple in the management of severe abnormal heart rhythms, but for us, on that day, it seemed heaven sent. And then, perhaps most miraculous of all, his "irreversible brain damage" wasn't really irreversible after all.

This lovely couple both retired, and married, five years after these events. They wintered in Florida and bought a second home there a year later. They traveled the world, and he joined several barbershop quartet singing groups. He had the profound blessing of living to see three grandsons join the family, and to see his second son engaged. Then one day, eleven years after our story began, he quite suddenly felt dizzy for a few seconds and collapsed. He was gone, from a large brain hemorrhage. His manner of passing is one I'd venture to say many of us would choose for ourselves.

I've spoken with his wife since then, and she tells me that he always referred to those eleven years as his "bonus" time, and that he and she were very grateful to have had them together.

And I'm very grateful I was such a "stubborn" ER doc that day, and that the stars aligned just the way they did.

DATE OF EVENT: JULY 2008

Please, God, I Have So Much More to Do

Benjamin Honigman, MD

As emergency physicians, we begin to form a mental picture of patients as soon as we get the ambulance call, well before the patient actually arrives in our emergency department. The typical image of a patient who has had a cardiac arrest is an older man, overweight, with a history of high blood pressure, smoking, and a sedentary lifestyle. Never did we imagine the ambulance bringing a buff eighteen-year-old football player from a local high school, a hometown hero who had already secured academic scholarships to college and hoped to also play football at a Big Ten university.

The young man was working out with his high school's track team to stay in shape for his upcoming football season. After a vigorous workout in ninety-degree heat, which was his norm, he passed out. A classmate who was the first one to notice him lying face down on the grass saw that he was not breathing. He screamed for help and two coaches responded. Not only had he stopped breathing but he also had no pulse: a true cardiac arrest. How could this be—a star athlete in great physical condition?

But this was not destined to be his time to die. One of the coaches, a medical technician, began chest compressions and the other coach began mouth-to-mouth breathing. The second coach, retelling the events for a newspaper reporter, said of his player in no uncertain terms, "He was dead," and remembers whispering between resuscitation breaths: "No. No. No. You're not going out like this." The young man's high school friend who was standing nearby told the reporter he prayed silently as well: "Lord, don't let him die. He's got a future. He never gives up. He's a good person. He's a role model."

Because of his coaches' heroism and skill, and the good fortune that they were present and knew exactly what to do when he went down, our patient started breathing again just as the paramedics and ambulance arrived.

The ambulance crew rapidly inserted an IV line (a tube for fluids and medicines) into his vein, placed him on a gurney, and lifted him into the back of the ambulance. He recalled praying in the ambulance as it sped away, "Please, God, I have so much more to do." Moments later, his heart started beating erratically and he had to be shocked with electricity en route to the hospital to regain a normal heartbeat. Once again the skill of those around him saved his life.

Our young football star arrived at the emergency department in dire shape, with severe oxygen deficiency. His lungs had filled up with fluid, a potentially fatal condition called pulmonary edema, and he was nearly choking on the pink frothy liquid that was coming from his lungs. It was clear that he was fighting for his breaths and fighting for his life.

We recognized that this was no routine cardiac arrest. Such an event in a fit young person requires immediate investigation for a congenital heart abnormality, something he might have been born with but didn't cause problems until now. While we were waiting for the heart specialist to arrive, our patient asked me through his labored breaths whether he had *HOCUM*. HOCUM is an acronym for *hypertrophic cardiomyopathy*, an affliction that causes an enlarged heart and takes the lives of many young people, especially athletes after exertion. I remember being taken aback by the insightfulness of his question, particularly coming at a time when he was struggling to breathe. How did he know about HOCUM? Our patient was clearly an aware and bright young man who had read tragic stories about young athletes dying on their playing fields. I believe he was trying to help us help him by suggesting a diagnosis, making sure we were thinking about heart conditions that are present at birth. HOCUM was certainly one of the abnormalities we had thought about, but we wouldn't know until the heart specialists could do their sophisticated testing.

We used medications to treat the excess fluid in his lungs and rapidly transported him to the cardiac catheterization lab, where the heart doctors could do their specialized tests. These studies showed that he did not have HOCUM, but rather had been born with another type of heart abnormality. In his case, one of the heart arteries, the left coronary, opened into the aorta (the main artery of the body) in the wrong position. This location created pressure and cut off some of the blood supply to the heart. Our patient was rushed to the operating room, where he had an open heart procedure to correct the placement of this artery into a normal position.

He could have died at each step along the way that day. From the track where he collapsed, to the ambulance where he developed a potentially fatal heart rhythm, to the emergency department where the fluid in his lungs threatened to suffocate him, to the heart catheterization lab and the operating room where potentially life-threatening emergency procedures were undertaken. Perhaps, as his coach had concluded, he even had died at one or more of those moments. But miraculously, at each of those stages, he seemed to have a guardian angel at his side directing skilled individuals who were at exactly the right place at exactly the right time to save his life. Why did his heart finally give out that particular day, near coaches skilled in CPR? Our young athlete had exerted himself on many occasions prior to this with no difficulty, often in workouts when no one was around. Why did tragedy not strike on a day when no one was around?

We later learned more about his background and the odds he had already beaten to even get to this point in his life. Our patient grew up in a poor home with the threat of gangs to deal with along the way. He had lived in foster homes and at one point in a homeless shelter. He became interested in sports and school and had outstanding mentors who cared deeply about him, guardian angels even before that fateful day on the track.

In his speech at his high-school graduation ceremony, our college-bound senior, the hometown hero, said: "There's no such thing as a self-made individual. You do as much as you can, but you can't do it all by yourself."

For the complete newspaper story from which some of the details and quotes were taken, see:

"Lord, don't let him die." J. Bunch, *Denver Post*, July 18, 2008; *http://www.denverpost.com/ci_9916358*

DATE OF EVENT: 2015

A Bona Fide Miracle

Jeremy Garrett, MD

Teenagers make choices and take chances—some of them unwise. That's what teenagers do. But on an unseasonably warm January day in the middle of a freezing winter, fourteen-year-old John Smith and two of his friends almost made their last choice ever. They decided to walk out on an icy lake.

At first things seemed great as the three posed for an impromptu picture with John's cell phone that went straight to social media. In an instant, their joy turned into terror when, moments after taking the photo, the ice gave way and all three boys plunged into the frigid water. The boys struggled to hang on to the crumbling icy ledge. One of the boys eventually managed to crawl out onto the surface; the other two clung to the ledge as best they could. One was able to make it until help arrived, but the other, John, lost his grip and eventually went under. He remained underwater for fifteen minutes.

When the rescue crew arrived, they at first didn't even know John was there. After rescuing his two friends, they donned protective gear, entered the water and began a search for John, probing the lake bottom with long blunt poles. Only days earlier, this same first-responder team had completed their ice-water rescue training. Miraculously, one specially trained paramedic felt a telltale thump with his probe; it was John. They acted quickly and retrieved the teen from the water. He was completely limp as they dragged him across the ice to shore, where they initiated cardiopulmonary resuscitation (CPR). Time was of the essence and they desperately continued CPR for fifteen minutes while transporting him to a local emergency room.

There, CPR continued with aggressive warming efforts for nearly a half hour longer, without response. As John remained pulseless, blue, without signs of life for well over an hour, doctors were about to stop resuscitative efforts and called his mother to the boy's side. As she prayed loudly and fervently, inexplicably his heart started beating on its own. While spontaneous circulation had resumed, no other signs of normal organ function were present.

John was then transferred to our pediatric intensive care unit. Upon arrival nearly three hours after the accident, profound circulatory shock (inadequate blood circulation and blood pressure) and multisystem organ failure persisted. He remained comatose with no brain activity or neurological activity present. We expected the worst. Despite his miraculous rescue and resuscitation, prospects for John's survival were discouragingly slim.

As is typical after a prolonged period without adequate blood and oxygen circulation, acid builds up in the body's tissues and threatens to keep vital organs shut down. Damage to John's organs and tissues was so severe his muscle cells were literally breaking open and dumping their contents into his bloodstream. After monitoring him carefully, treating his acid buildup, continuing a state of induced hypothermia (keeping his body temperature low), working hard to prevent kidney failure, providing supplemental oxygen with maximum settings on a ventilator (breathing machine), and supporting circulation for the next sixteen hours, a glimmer of hope began to return. We became confident his body would survive. But even with his heart re-started and his vital organs now finally being supplied with blood, little hope remained that he could recover his brain function after such prolonged sub-mersion requiring such protracted CPR.

Although there are many stories of cold water drowning with surpris-ingly good outcomes, those require a special combination of factors—none of which were present for John except the cold water—and even that wasn't optimal. Ideally, to preserve brain function, the water must be cold enough to chill the brain before the blood circulation to the brain stops. In this case, the lake temperature was not low enough, and John's body size much larger than the typical survival case, so blood flow to his brain would have almost certainly stopped before his brain chilled to a temperature that might be pro-tective. While his body temperature on arrival in the emergency room was a life-threateningly low 88 degrees Fahrenheit, we had no reason to believe it got that low in the proper sequence needed to preserve brain function.

But I was wrong—and I was never so glad about it.

Within forty-eight hours of arrival to our unit, John began opening his eyes. Shortly after that, with the breathing tube still in his throat, he began answering complex questions I asked about his two favorite professional bas-ketball players. Using his hands, John gave the answers—left hand for LeBron James, right hand for Michael Jordan. When he answered all the questions correctly, I knew he would recover his brain function.

I had never seen anything this astonishing in over twenty-five years of doing intensive care medicine.

After a week on the ventilator and sixteen days of hospital care, John went home, continuing to receive physical therapy to regain fine motor movements in his hands. His brain function was otherwise entirely normal. When the media interviewed his parents and the doctors and nurses in the emergency room where John was first taken, with one voice they all declared that John's heartbeat starting right after his mother's prayer was a miracle. Because I'd cared for him at our facility for many days afterward, the news media also interviewed me. I called his brain recovery a bona fide miracle. This is not hyperbole—there were really no other words to describe it.

Nothing has happened to change my mind since. After his release from the hospital, John eventually went back to school after missing many weeks, caught up with his studies, graduated middle school with his friends, returned to playing basketball and, incredibly, is fully back to being an active teenager.

DATE OF EVENT: SEPTEMBER 2014

She Pointed Up to Heaven

Michael Fleischer, MD

In residency training, young doctors speak of "white clouds" and "black clouds." Residents with "black clouds" are the ones with tough, sleepless nights on call, their patients "crashing" with complications and bad outcomes. Doctors with "white clouds" rarely have things go wrong on their watch. I had the reputation among my fellow residents of having a "white cloud." I'll leave it to you to decide whether, on this September morning, long past my residency days, I had a white cloud or a black cloud over my head. I know what I would call it.

I was on my way to the hospital to do a routine repeat caesarean section on Ruby at thirty-nine weeks (full term) of pregnancy. I had delivered her previous baby seven years earlier, also by C-section due to Ruby's high blood pressure. Ruby remained on blood pressure medicine throughout this current pregnancy, with stable pressures throughout an otherwise uncomplicated pregnancy.

I was in a good mood because it was my half day on call, and I knew I could go home after the procedure and rest. I had been under the weather all weekend and was finally starting to feel better and no longer contagious, but a short day would help a lot. I greeted Ruby and her family in the pre-op area. They were very excited to see me since they knew that I had been ill, and they thought I might not be able to do her surgery. Ruby and her sister spoke English; however, the rest of the family spoke only Portuguese.

After checking her vital signs, labs, and the fetal heart tracing, I helped the nurses take Ruby to the operating room. Her spinal anesthesia injection went in easily, and we began the surgery. A few minutes later I delivered a healthy baby boy and everybody was very happy and excited. Her husband hurried over to cut the cord. Within fifteen minutes, the surgery was over, the incision closed, and Ruby was taken to the recovery room.

I returned to the family in the waiting area to tell them the good news that everything went well and the baby was healthy. They would be allowed in to see Ruby in a little while. I left the area to round on my other patients before heading home.

That's when everything went downhill fast. My beeper sounded simultaneously to hearing my name being called urgently overhead on the hospital loudspeaker—always a bad sign. I found my patient back on the operating room table with a breathing tube inserted in her windpipe. The anesthesiologist informed me that Ruby had stopped breathing in the recovery room. Thankfully, he was right there at the time and quickly inserted the tube. Her blood pressure was now unstable, dangerously low. I carefully assessed Ruby. She was not bleeding from her incision or from her vagina. Her urine output was adequate. I used an ultrasound test to see if there was blood in her abdomen; there was not. Everything from the surgery was intact. I knew her sudden respiratory (breathing) arrest was either due to a pulmonary embolism or an amniotic fluid embolism; neither would be good news, but the first one is much more treatable than the second one. A pulmonary embolism is a blood clot that has spread from the lower part of the body to the lungs, where it can cause chest pain, difficulty breathing, and even a total respiratory or cardiac arrest. An amniotic fluid embolism is a much more rare condition where the fluid that surrounds the baby in the womb enters the mother's bloodstream. This is a highly lethal condition, killing as many as 60 to 80 percent of women who develop it, and it often causes brain damage in survivors. Typically, hospital stays of weeks or even months are required following amniotic fluid embolism.

The anesthesiologist continued to assist Ruby's breathing as well as give her strong medicines to keep her blood pressure from falling. Doctors specializing in intensive care arrived to help as well. At this point, I knew I had to discuss the situation with the family. We had been working to stabilize Ruby's blood pressures for at least thirty minutes. I spoke with her sister, who translated everything for Ruby's husband and family. I explained that Ruby had difficulty breathing, and we were struggling to get her vital signs under control so that we could take her to the radiology suite for special X-ray testing to determine the problem. If testing found a pulmonary embolism was threatening her life, we may be able to retrieve the clot from the lungs using a special catheter (tube) and she would be fine. On the other hand, if we determine it was an amniotic fluid embolism ... well, that might be a very different story. They understood and would wait patiently.

I returned to Ruby's side as we monitored her vital signs and electrocardiogram (EKG). Despite the strong medicines we were giving her, we still could not maintain an adequate blood pressure, now two hours into her crisis. That's when we saw it on the monitor—she no longer had a regular heartbeat. In fact, she no longer had a heartbeat at all! Ruby was in cardiac arrest! We immediately started cardiopulmonary resuscitation (CPR). The intensive care specialist was the first to begin pumping on Ruby's chest, counting one, two, three, four, five, six, seven, eight, nine, ten. Oxygen was flowing into her lungs from the breathing tube, but heart compressions were essential to circulate the oxygen to the brain and other vital organs. He continued the exhausting pumping, then asked for someone else to help. The anesthesiologist took over.

A little while later, it was my turn to pump her chest. I couldn't believe what I was witnessing. My routine C-section had turned into a tragedy. She was going to die. My patient—this mom, wife, sister, and daughter—was about to die on my watch. All we could do was continue CPR and desperately try to maintain her blood pressure.

I spoke to the family again. I explained the catastrophic turn of events and how the likelihood of survival was very low. I told them that we would do everything we could, and I then returned to the OR. We continued CPR for another thirty minutes. Nothing changed. We shocked her with the defibrillator paddles hoping to jump-start her heart, medicated her with drugs intended to stimulate the heart, and continued compressions. And then we repeated the steps over and over again.

Ultimately, it became obvious to all of us that the time had come for the family to say good-bye. We wanted them to be able to talk to her, hug her, and kiss her before she was officially pronounced "dead," although after forty-five minutes without a pulse and nearly three hours without adequate blood pressure, she was already, for all intents and purposes, gone. We also wanted the family to see the many people working so hard to resuscitate Ruby so they would know we were doing everything humanly possible to save her.

As Ruby's family filed into the OR where we were still working feverishly, they screamed out her name in anguish. They shouted their love for her. They cried out that it was not her time. They pleaded with God not to take her. Her mother asked God to take her instead. It was beyond emotional, it was heart-wrenching. I continued chest compressions while the family hugged and kissed her. Once they each had a chance to say tearful good-byes, they gathered in the waiting room. I joined them as we huddled closely and said a prayer. Then I returned to Ruby.

We had performed CPR for well over forty-five minutes with no response. We had shocked her five times and given her multiple rounds of medicines. There was nothing left to do. We stopped our compressions and just watched the heart monitor. We kept the tube in her windpipe because her EKG showed some type of vague background electrical activity, although no true beats. We waited for it to stop completely before pulling the tube out. We waited for the flat line.

Then the impossible happened. A blip of a beat on the monitor. Then another. Then another. Somehow, Ruby's heart started to pump on its own, now with a normal rhythm. And just as impossibly, her blood pressure was suddenly normal. It seemed she would be okay. Would she, actually? After no heartbeat for more than forty-five minutes and without a normal blood pressure for nearly three hours, how would her brain function? What other organ damage might she have sustained? Kidneys? Heart? What type of life would she have if she survived? At this point, we couldn't answer those questions or be distracted by them. For now, she was alive! We told the family. In unison they screamed for joy and rushed back into the OR. They proclaimed their faith that God exists and began praying out loud.

We gave them some time with Ruby and then took her to the radiology suite. We still had to determine if she had a pulmonary embolism as the cause of all of this and whether we could remove it. Unfortunately, the scan did not reveal a pulmonary embolism, meaning she definitely had an amniotic fluid embolism. We took her to the intensive care unit to monitor her for the dread complications of this condition, anticipating a long and difficult stay there. For now, at least, she was stable. I couldn't do anything more at this point so I went home, exhausted and numb, leaving her in the good hands of the intensive care doctors.

I was not even halfway home when the nurse called me with unimaginably wonderful news. Ruby opened her eyes! She responded to questions by nodding her head. She pointed up to heaven. She knew she was okay. I couldn't believe it. Ruby's only bump in the road from there was an episode of bleeding from the incision site, which I was able to stop with a couple of stitches. The next day I sat with Ruby and explained everything that had happened, barely believing my own words. Later that day, we were able to safely remove the breathing tube, confident she was out of the woods. No brain damage, no other organ damage, no broken ribs despite all the pounding on her chest—she didn't even have bruising.

Defying all the statistics and all the textbooks, three days later Ruby went home with her healthy baby and entire family. I think about this day very often. Was it God? The prayers of her family? Was it luck? Was it the skill of the medical team? Was all of this evidence of a black cloud or a white cloud over my head? I choose white.

4

Extraordinary Awakenings

Severe impairment of brain function leaves patients and their families in medical and emotional limbo. Coma can result from many causes, but the longer it lasts, the worse the prognosis.

These essays describe patients in prolonged coma following severe brain injuries from infections, shock, stroke, medication error, and drowning. As the days and weeks wore on, their families were told there was little to no hope for improvement. Brain death and a vegetative state seemed certain.

Yet, right before our eyes, these patients opened theirs.

A Miraculous Smile

Rodney E. Willoughby, MD

I was in training as a pediatrician in a busy children's hospital with far too many patients to care for. My responsibilities included a ward where children were rehabilitated after serious injuries. Most did not recover fully. Many were connected to breathing machines through tubes inserted directly through the skin in their necks. It was a sad place.

Heather was a thirteen-year-old with severe asthma who had been at summer camp in July. She developed walking pneumonia and was prescribed an antibiotic to treat her infection. Unfortunately, the camp doctor didn't realize that particular antibiotic interacted with her asthma medication, increasing her blood levels of the asthma medicine to toxic levels. As a result, Heather had a seizure, vomited, choked on her vomit, and stopped breathing. She was found unresponsive and was airlifted to our hospital. She did not recover meaningful activity. She had been in a coma for four months. She was fed through a tube into her stomach. Her mother visited every day and made sure she was always clean and well-groomed.

Heather developed a fever and I was called to look her over for a possible infection. In medical school, we are taught to treat patients with respect. We are supposed to inform patients what we are doing to them and why. This lesson is emphasized even in the extreme, such as when patients are unconscious. We are regaled in school with stories of patients (usually doctors themselves, who at one time were under treatment and recovered) recalling what was said about them by others at bedside when they were thought to be unconscious. Patients who couldn't move after trauma or stroke but who were fully conscious, in pain, and hearing every word, retold their agonizing experiences to us. But, when you are very busy and very tired, it is easy to take the shortcut and not bother with such niceties as fully informing and showing respect to a girl in coma for many months. After all, there is almost no hope after so long.

Dutifully, but with some internal skepticism about how necessary it was, I warned Heather about my cold stethoscope and warned her again when I was about to push on her belly as part of my exam. I next told her that I would look in her ears. I had just heard a great joke from the head nurse on another ward—one of those that make you smile for the rest of the day. I decided to tell Heather the joke while at her ear; the joke would just be between the two of us.

To my amazement, she smiled! I know because I was going to examine her mouth next, and the smile was still there as I got my tongue blade ready. So now I didn't know what to do. Was it just a random grimace? I am terrible at jokes because I can never remember them. I had no other jokes ready. I resolved to get another joke from my friendly nurse and try again the next day.

Heather's mother was there when I next came by. I was embarrassed to try out my new joke in front of such a large audience (two, one of them comatose), and I was worried about creating false hope in her mother. I decided to try my joke, but only after procrastinating through my entire examination. Again, on cue, Heather smiled. Her mother saw it immediately and was so overjoyed that she started crying. I told her mother about the previous day and suggested she buy a book of jokes as my reserves were spent.

Over the next week, the positive signs kept coming, leaving no doubt that Heather was, indeed, making significant progress. She smiled at some but not all jokes (probably a good sign), opened her eyes, and began to nod yes or no when I asked her questions. She seemed to have a crush on one of the male doctors. She was discharged home a few weeks later—now walking and talking on the way to a full recovery.

Since that experience early in my career, I always talk to my sedated or unresponsive patients, without questioning its necessity or value. I even tell a joke or two.

DATE OF EVENT: 1974

As if Nothing Much Had Ever Happened

Alan R. Spitzer, MD

Near the end of my second year of pediatrics residency, I was assigned to the pediatric intensive care unit (PICU) of one of the foremost children's hospitals in the country. Patients admitted to the PICU were always difficult management problems and often extremely ill. Needless to say, as a young resident-in-training, my anxiety each and every day during this rotation was significant.

During the second week of the rotation, I was on call one night when I received a page from the senior resident notifying me that a young child was being admitted to my service who was becoming progressively *obtunded* (losing consciousness, difficult to arouse). Upon learning that the boy was approximately two years of age, I initially assumed it was going to be some type of ingestion of a toxic material that would need sorting out and immediate therapy. Toddlers tend to get into dangerous chemicals like cleaning fluids, pesticides, cosmetics, or their parents' medicines and end up in PICUs around the country every day. This child was accompanied to the PICU by his parents, who told me he was never out of their sight and it was not possible he had ingested anything. I also learned from them that Michael (not his real name) had been running a moderate fever for about twenty-four hours, which they assumed was probably due to a developing cold. He and his two older siblings were always sharing their germs and getting each other sick. Earlier in the day, he had been very irritable and fussy, refusing to eat and crying almost constantly. Shortly after dinner, his irritability diminished, but

Michael had now become progressively sleepier to the point where it was difficult to awaken him. His parents became concerned and brought him to our emergency room for evaluation, and from there he was subsequently admitted to the PICU.

I told the family that I would like to examine Michael and I might have further questions for them after I did his physical exam. They told me they would be here all night with him, as they had dropped their other two children off at their grandparents' house. At that point, I turned to the child on the bed and I was immediately taken aback by his appearance. Not only was this child acutely ill, but his physical appearance resembled that of my own son, Stephen, so closely that I had to look twice to reassure myself that this was, in fact, another child and not my son. Michael's hair color, skin color, and physical build were nearly identical to my son's, and when I checked his birth date, he was born just a few weeks before my son. Pediatricians often say that one of the toughest parts of our job is that we "project" our own children onto our patients, sometimes identifying so strongly with their parents that it's difficult to stay objective for the medical issues we have to confront. However, this was even worse—Michael more than just reminded me of my son, he looked just like him!

I could hardly imagine the profound anxiety that this family had to be going through to witness such a sudden, dramatic deterioration right before their eyes. On the remainder of Michael's physical exam, in addition to the obtundation, I discovered he had significant stiffness of the back and spine, pointing to either meningitis (a bacterial infection of the covering of the brain) or encephalitis (a viral infection of the brain itself) as the most likely diagnoses. I sent blood tests to the lab and performed a spinal tap, inserting a needle between the vertebral bones of the spine to withdraw a small amount of the fluid that bathes the brain and spinal cord for additional tests. We began intravenous (directly into a vein) therapy with fluids and antibiotics. The blood tests confirmed there had been no ingestion, and the spinal fluid tests indicated encephalitis was the more probable cause. Some days later, a diagnosis of *Eastern equine encephalitis* (EEE) was confirmed. EEE is a rare brain infection caused by a virus and transmitted by the bite of a mosquito. It has the most serious consequences; the Centers for Disease Control and Prevention (CDC) reports that about one-third of patients die, and the majority of survivors are left with significant brain damage. Other than providing support for breathing, hydration, seizures, and brain swelling, there was nothing else we could do. To this day there is still no specific treatment for this infection; antibiotics don't work against viral infections like this.

Michael's initial hospital course was very stormy, with seizures, respiratory insufficiency (inability to breathe adequately) that required a breathing machine, and intermittent cardiovascular instability (an irregular and weak heartbeat). Each and every time I looked at this unfortunate child, who looked so much like my son, I became distraught, frantic with the desire to somehow make him well again. For his parents, I could not do enough, yet whatever I did never seemed adequate to me for what they were going through. Finally, after a few extremely difficult days when death always seemed but one step away, his condition stabilized and we were able to begin removing some of his acute life support equipment.

Unfortunately, although his body functions stabilized, he remained comatose. The supervising physician and I finally had to inform his family that, given the known history of this terrible disease, it was likely that Michael had suffered significant brain injury and would need supportive care for the remainder of his life. I could not imagine the grief that this family must have felt, nor could I envision how I would respond if those words were told to me about my own son. After another week, we made the decision, with his parents, to transfer Michael to our affiliated long-term care hospital where his needs could be better met and some planning undertaken with the family for the child's grim-looking future.

I vividly recall as he left the PICU having a sense of profound failure. Yes, we had saved his life, but to what end? And for months afterward, each time I looked at my own son, I was so grateful for his good health, but I could never stop thinking about Michael. I would occasionally call and inquire about him, but the message was always the same—no change. Eventually, the nonstop bombardment of new responsibilities and new patients that befall a physician-in-training intervened and this boy faded somewhat from my mind, though he was never very far away. At moments of happiness and contentment at home with my own son, my thoughts inevitably drifted to Michael and his parents.

One day while walking through the hallway, I bumped into one of the PICU nurses who had cared for Michael during his stay with us. "Remember the boy with the Eastern equine encephalitis from a few months ago?" she remarked.

"Sure," I said, "I'll never forget him."

"Well, then," she beamed, "you'll be pleased to know he apparently woke up this morning and said that he was hungry!"

I could not believe it. I rushed to find someone to cover for me and drove to the long-term care hospital. There I found Michael and his parents, the family overwhelmed with joy, tears flowing freely. He sat in his mother's arms, sucking his thumb, and looking for all the world as if nothing much had ever happened, testimony to the superb nursing care that accompanied him throughout his illness. It was very difficult for me to control my own emotions, but I was thrilled beyond words. His miraculous awakening made it feel as if, once again, all was right with the world.

I saw Michael in clinic for follow-up for the next year with the neurology team, but his development, after a bit of a lag, soon proceeded apace and he rapidly caught up in his milestones. He didn't need specialists any longer. His family decided to get his ongoing care from his own pediatrician, the true goal for all of us caring for the sickest of patients.

I never saw Michael again, but this experience has never left me. It reminds me to never give up hope when there is even a glimmer that something remarkable might take place. And to this day, when I look with pride at my son Stephen, now an adult with his own kids, I hope that Michael has rewarded his family with the same sense of joy that Stephen has always given me.

For more on EEE, see: *http://www.cdc.gov/easternequineencephalitis/*

DATE OF EVENT: AUGUST–SEPTEMBER 1977

A Blonde Blur

John W. Ogle, MD

She had been a previously healthy blonde two-year-old described by her parents as full of energy and the spark of life. She contracted a serious disease called *hemolytic uremic syndrome* in which a patient's kidneys can gradually fail, and hers did. The disease is poorly understood, but the treatment requires dialysis to filter the blood from toxins until the kidneys hopefully recover. But the usually routine procedure to place a catheter for dialysis had complications and she went into shock, severely dropping her blood pressure. As a consequence of the shock she suffered a profound injury to her brain.

I assumed her care as she transferred out of the intensive care unit. She had almost no normal neurological findings: she did not move voluntarily, could not speak, and could not eat or drink. In response to touch and voice, she went into painful spasms. She was in deep coma and responded neither to her parents nor to her doctors. She had frequent seizures and had to be fed through a tube passed from her nose into her stomach. Ironically, although her brain was devastated by the procedure to treat her kidneys, they began working better. She developed many more complications, including severe stomach and intestinal bleeding and pneumonia. She needed transfusions, a tube in her chest, and frequent medications for elevated blood pressure. For weeks there seemed to be daily medical crises.

Her parents were told that their beautiful daughter's brain would likely never recover from her injury and that she would continue in coma and eventually succumb to a seizure or an infection such as pneumonia. They politely and stoically heard all of the predictions and tried to cope with the implications. They were very attentive to their daughter, but very private, holding all of the staff at a bit of a distance. Remaining very persistent in their belief their daughter would recover, her parents were certain she just needed more time. Their questions for the neurologists were thoughtful and to the point, but they declined doctors' suggestions for surgeries that would make their child's breathing and feeding in a long-term care facility easier—they insisted on taking her home and providing her daily care themselves, in her own bedroom. They were willing to accept the consequences of whatever happened next.

This was my first year as a pediatrics resident-in-training. I had little experience with this type of case or with a family that declined physician recommendations for care. The neurology specialists, whose job it is to assess brain damage, commented on the highly unrealistic expectations of the family for their daughter's recovery. Her parents expressed appreciation that I never questioned their decision to take their daughter home. As the parents requested, and with serious reservations about the wisdom of their decision, we sent her home; it was September. The nature of training being what it is, I went on to other clinics, wards, and hospitals, but I frequently wondered what happened to this little girl. Had she died as predicted? Had her parents given up on her recovery? Was she in a long-term care facility?

About four months later, I was working on the morning of December 24—Christmas Eve—when I was greeted by the parents, who had returned to the hospital for a routine follow-up appointment with the kidney specialists. I did not recognize their gorgeous daughter, a blonde blur who came running down the hall. She had bitten off the tip of her tongue during one of her seizures in the intensive care unit months ago, and her "s" sound came out with a little hiss. She was otherwise the perfect spark of life her parents had described before any of this had started. I was too shocked to ask them about any of the details of their daughter's recovery, and I never saw them again. I would love to know how that little blonde blur is doing now.

This is such a vivid memory for me, I can still "see" this child as if she were running down the hall toward me today. December 24 was the day I discovered miracles. To this day, I think about her frequently as I care for other difficult cases, whenever parents are hoping for their own miracle.

DATE OF EVENT: 1972 OR 1973

The Lazarus Child

Mary P. Glode, MD

I was a pediatrics intern in a large Southern city, when a previously healthy nine-year-old boy was admitted to the hospital with *encephalitis*, a very serious infection of the brain. We did every test we knew about at the time to try and discover the cause of his infection, but no cause was found. He stopped talking, stopped eating, and lapsed into a deep coma. We were all devastated that we could do nothing to help this child. We asked the chairman of the pediatrics department to please come see the boy with us. The chairman was a brilliant doctor, the person to whom we turned with the most difficult cases—he usually was able to come up with an answer and a plan. He reviewed the case and carefully examined the child, but could only reassure us that we had done everything we could, and there was nothing more that could be done. It was clear to all of us that our chairman did not think this child would recover from his coma.

Each day, we carefully assessed the child, examining him and reviewing the blood tests and brain scans, but he remained deeply comatose for weeks. We observed no apparent progress in his condition, and we were no closer to understanding the cause of the child's illness. Then one day everything changed. It was a spring morning, many weeks after the boy had been admitted to the hospital. As we entered his room on rounds, the child suddenly opened his eyes and said quite clearly, "I'm hungry, can I have a hamburger?"

We were absolutely stunned. There had been no progress on rounds as recently as the night before. Ecstatic, we called the child's mother, who was still at home that morning (since we made rounds quite early). Our next call was to our department chairman to tell him the wonderful news. He immediately came to see the boy and was speechless, but thrilled, also without an explanation for the child's astonishing turnaround.

The little boy recovered completely over a period of several months and had no memory of his illness. In the years since, I have always referred to this case as the "Lazarus child" since it seemed to me that he had come back from death.

DATE OF EVENT: FEBRUARY 2002

A Mother's Voice, a Husband's Devotion, a Patient's Courage

Anthony Suchman, MD, MA

Mary Clark (not her real name) was a friend of my artist wife, Lynne, long before she became my patient. Mary was an engaged and creative guidance counselor in an urban public middle school and was well along her intended path to earn her doctorate and become a school principal. She and Lynne became friends when, in response to a racially charged altercation in the school cafeteria, they engaged more than sixty students in a large art project: creating murals for the school's atrium that depicted their communities. They then developed a student-run business selling T-shirts, carry bags, and greeting cards bearing photographic reproductions of the murals and, with the help of several teachers, developed an entire sixth-grade curriculum around the business. As I said, Mary was engaged and creative, a beacon of light to her school, her family and friends, and her whole community.

One Friday, Mary started to feel unwell with body aches, a headache, and general fatigue. She called her doctor's office and was advised to take a pain reliever, which helped temporarily. But by Monday her headache was steadily worsening. That evening, right in the middle of giving a presentation to her graduate school class, she felt so sick she had to excuse herself. She went out in the hall, fell, tried to get up, and lost consciousness. At the age of forty-two, Mary's light had suddenly been all but snuffed out by an enormous stroke.

It turned out that Mary had *vasculitis*, inflammation of the blood vessels of her brain due to a disease called *systemic lupus erythematosus* (or *lupus*). The vasculitis damaged the blood vessel walls and made them weak. A large vessel had ruptured, resulting in the formation of an orange-sized pool of blood in her head that squeezed and distorted most of her brain. Mary was not brain-dead; part of her brainstem (which attends to basic tasks of body regulation) was still functioning but she was in a dense coma, completely unresponsive to her surroundings.

The doctors told Mary's husband, James, that her chances of recovery were around 5 percent. As he told me later, he simply refused to believe that. Every night he stayed with her in the hospital, talking to her and encouraging her. He made sure that her hands, arms, feet, and legs were moved through their full range of motion every day to maintain their suppleness and flexibility, and to prevent the development of muscle contractures. But week after week, her outlook dimmed as she showed no sign of awareness and made no spontaneous movements. Still, he never stopped believing and the hospital staff never stopped supporting him in his hope. He read everything he could find about stroke and investigated all the latest experimental therapies.

One day, after Mary had been in the hospital for five weeks with no change in her condition, her mother called James to see how things were going, as she often did. It occurred to James to hold the telephone up to Mary's ear; maybe her mother's voice would rouse her. *Why not? Let's try anything*, he thought. To everyone's astonishment, when her mother said, "Hello," Mary mumbled hello right back.

And with that Mary woke up. She had no idea how much time had elapsed. But she did know she couldn't move her right arm or leg. And she couldn't make her mouth speak, though she knew exactly what she wanted to say and could comprehend everything that other people said to her. It didn't take her long to understand what had happened; she was determined to work her way back.

And work she did. Over the ensuing weeks, months, and years she applied herself full-bore to her physical, occupational, and speech therapy. James was always right there with her; he even fashioned a physical therapy gym for her at home so she could exercise more. She and James took encouragement from every gain, no matter how small, and then worked for more. James continued to read voraciously and found a variety of assistive devices and novel therapies. By then I had become Mary's primary care physician; we all reviewed his discoveries and decided together which ones to pursue.

Mary's family and friends provided steadfast support, too. While Mary was in rehab, James created a schedule so that someone—a family member or friend—would be with her at all times. After Mary went home from rehab, knowing how much she enjoyed art, her friends arranged for her to spend time each week in Lynne's art studio. At first Mary just enjoyed being in that environment; she was unable to make anything. But then a weaver helped her learn to push the shuttle through the warp to make simple weavings. Then she was able to scribble, then draw, then paint. In her first visits she would arrive in a wheelchair, driven by a home health aide. Then she walked in with a walker, then with a cane, and finally without any assistive device, having driven to the studio by herself.

For three years after her stroke Mary continued to make progress. In addition to walking and driving she regained partial use of her right arm and much of her speech, though not to the point of full fluency. When words and phrases elude her, she waves it off with a chuckle and finds other ways to make her thoughts known.

As it became clear that she would not be able to resume her career in education, Mary let go of her identity as an educator and claimed a new one—artist—which she finds even more fulfilling. What started as recreation and socialization has become her vocation. Sharing studio space with Lynne, she has become quite accomplished, mastering the complex cutting, pasting, and painting of fabric collage and developing a fine eye and original vision in her work. Mary lives on her own in Florida for several months each year to escape the threat of winter ice while James works and holds down the fort at home. And, as I write these words, she and James have traveled to the South to attend the birth of their first grandchild. Mary regards every aspect of her life as a blessing; she would change nothing.

There are many miracles here. One is, of course, the physical one: that such an enormous blood clot could break down and be reabsorbed little by little, making room for Mary's brain to re-expand, and that as squeezed and distorted as it was for so many weeks, her brain did not sustain more extensive permanent damage. Then there's the miracle of awakening to a mother's voice. Another is James' unwavering belief and devotion. While we can't know if his belief influenced the course of Mary's blood clot, James' tireless advocacy certainly contributed to her remarkable functional improvement, as did the deep and sustained support of family and friends. Finally, Mary's courage, determination, resilience, and humor in the face of overwhelming odds were miraculous in their own right.

Her spirit is now as bright as ever, not only shining on her friends and family but also lighting a path for others as she helps other stroke survivors as a peer counselor. For all these reasons, Mary's is one of the most inspiring recoveries I've ever witnessed.

DATE OF EVENT: DECEMBER 1980

The Squeeze

Harley A. Rotbart, MD

I was a second-year pediatrics resident doing my intensive care unit (ICU) rotation at a large children's hospital. Two young brothers, ages three and seven, were brought into our emergency room and then the ICU after near-drowning episodes. It was winter, and the three-year-old had fallen into a swimming pool with enough residual water that he couldn't stand. His seven-year-old brother jumped in, pulled the younger boy to one of the pool's steps where the three-year-old's head was out of the water, but the seven-year-old was then himself overwhelmed by the freezing water and couldn't get out before submerging. When paramedics arrived, both boys were unconscious.

In the ICU, the younger boy regained consciousness within a few hours and was neurologically normal; he went home within a few days. The older brother remained in a coma for several weeks. The family stood vigil every day, and we, the residents, took over in the evenings and overnight, holding the older boy's hand, talking and singing to him. We all prayed. Not in an organized way, or even in a traditional way, but each of us in his or her own way. It was on my "watch," late at night when I felt the boy squeeze my hand while I was reading to him. Just one squeeze.

This was now weeks into his stay and, because there had been no progress, discussions were beginning in the ICU about discontinuing life support, brain death, and organ donation. I told everyone on rounds the next morning about the hand squeeze. Most of my colleagues and supervisors attributed it to involuntary muscle spasms. Indeed, medically, by all our measures of brain function and assessments of neurologic recovery, there was not even the slightest possibility that this child could have made a conscious effort to squeeze my hand. But then someone else also felt it after rounds that morning, and then again that afternoon, now in response to command. The child's parents were overwhelmed with joy and hope when they felt their son's hand squeeze for the first time. None of us knew quite what to make of it or how much to hope for.

It would be several more days before the boy opened his eyes; a few hours after that he smiled, still with a breathing tube in place. When he walked out of the hospital more than two months after the near-drowning and his heroic rescue of his little brother, we all cheered and cried. We had cried many times in the weeks preceding, and I still cry whenever I recall this story.

5

Unimaginable Disasters

Terrible things can happen to people in an instant. In the blink of an eye, life or limb may hang in the balance of disastrous events that could not possibly have been foreseen or even imagined. Freak accidents, catastrophic injuries, bolts of lightning, horrific acts of crime.

The stories in this chapter describe just such disastrous events, where hope for survival or meaningful recovery seemed futile.

DATE OF EVENT: DECEMBER 7, 2007

Free Fall: If You Are a Believer in Miracles, This Would Be One

Philip S. Barie, MD, MBA, Master CCM

People fall from the sky all the time, at least in New York City where I live and work. Construction workers; alleged criminals who fall from fire escapes trying to elude the authorities; troubled souls who jump—we have seen them all and cared for their injuries. There are so many skyscrapers, and even the "low-rise" buildings are often six to eight stories tall. As a general rule, people who fall three stories—thirty to thirty-six feet—have about a fifty-fifty chance of surviving. If they do survive it is a hard road to recovery. Weeks in the hospital and months of rehabilitation are in store, with no guarantee of being made whole. Falls from greater height, or from almost any height if they hit their heads and suffer a brain injury, carry a much worse prognosis.

In 2003, my colleagues and I published a paper in a respected medical journal describing the unlikely survival of a man who plunged from the nineteenth floor of a building. That case was remarkable, and worthy of publication for our colleagues in the field to read, because that man survived against all odds. Nearly 100 percent of those who fall ten stories are killed by the fall—they don't even survive long enough to reach the hospital. Survival after a nineteen-story fall? Extraordinary, indeed, and seemingly impossible. I have taken care of two people who survived twelve-story falls, one who survived a fourteen-story fall, and the patient we reported in the medical journal who survived the nineteen-story plunge. The chances of survival from that height are tiny—much less than 1 percent. He survived because he struck a tree branch about two stories above ground, breaking his fall before the limb itself broke and crashed to the ground with him, impaled in his back.

Little could I have known when we wrote of that man who fell nineteen stories that a few years later I would be privileged to be involved in a far more extraordinary and seemingly impossible survival story.

✧ ✧ ✧

December 7 is a profoundly sorrowful anniversary in American history—the day the United States naval base at Pearl Harbor in Hawaii was struck from a surprise attack by the Japanese, drawing our country into World War II. That morning in 2007 was the sixty-sixth anniversary of the surprise attack. The day dawned clear and cool, with scattered clouds and a slight breeze from the southwest. All in all not bad for December in New York City. Really nothing to foreshadow the horror about to unfold.

About 9:30 AM thirty-seven-year-old Alcides and his younger brother reported for work to wash the exterior windows of a modernistic high-rise residential tower on the Upper East Side of Manhattan, about fourteen blocks from the hospital where a life-and-death drama was about to unfold. Sheathed in black glass, the building stands forty-seven stories tall and looks like something out of a science-fiction movie. Everyone who lives or works in the neighborhood knows the building; its appearance is sleek and stark against the skyline, and it towers, literally, above every other building nearby.

As Alcides and his brother climbed over the roofline and lowered themselves onto their platform, all hell broke loose—literally. The platform broke from its moorings and plunged onto concrete below, killing Alcides' brother instantly and injuring Alcides grievously. In the aftermath, physicists estimated (the math is complex) that it took five to six seconds to fall from that height, speeding perhaps eighty miles per hour and still accelerating at impact. A fall from an "unsurvivable" height of more than 500 feet, at a high rate of speed, onto a concrete alleyway? And someone is still alive? Did the platform serve as a sort of parasail, slowing the descent? Pure speculation.

When the fire department first-responders arrived at the scene, they saw both tragedy and wonder. Alcides' brother's body was severed in half after landing on a fence in the alleyway, but Alcides was sitting upright on the aluminum window-washing platform, breathing, dazed, semi-conscious. The ambulance crew arrived and performed a "scoop and run," quickly and carefully lifting Alcides onto a gurney and speeding the fourteen city blocks (just under three-quarters of a mile) to our hospital.

When our trauma surgery team was called to the emergency department (ED) to await the ambulance carrying Alcides, I knew only that the patient was said to have fallen from atop a forty-seven-story building. *Wait . . . what? How is it possible that we are awaiting a living patient?* I thought. *Surely he would be declared dead on arrival, or it would be obvious there was little or nothing we could do.*

But we didn't know many of these details in real time, and there was little time to question what we heard, or to dwell on the details at such a moment. There would be time later to search the Internet for news reports that would fill the gaps in our knowledge and satisfy our curiosity. For the time being, we readied ourselves for whatever the ambulance would bring to us in about two minutes. Any reliable information is helpful to anticipate certain patterns of injury or complications, but so often in trauma we don't have reliable information. It could be because no one witnessed the event. When a patient is "found down," for instance, were they assaulted? Struck by a car in a hit-and-run? Or did a collapse arise from some medical problem such as a heart attack or stroke, leading to injury only secondarily? Sometimes, if criminality is involved, the information available may be intended to deceive ("I was minding my own business, when . . ."). So we train to integrate the information we have, and rely mostly on what our eyes, ears, and hands tell us from examining the patient. It will be several crucial minutes before the results of lab tests or X-rays become available. Trauma surgeons make rapid, momentous decisions every day, based on incomplete or even conflicting information. We must, or else a life may ebb away.

The doors to the ambulance flung open and the crew ran, at breakneck speed, the thirty-foot straight shot into our ED. Suppressing our disbelief, we set to work assessing the patient and beginning treatment. In trauma, diagnosis and therapy often have to occur simultaneously, processes known as *triage* and *resuscitation*. Alcides' face had barely a scratch, but that was misleading—the rest of his body was pulverized. He was comatose and having difficulty breathing, so a breathing tube was inserted in his windpipe and he was attached to a breathing machine. Intravenous catheters (tubes in his veins) were placed for administration of fluid and blood. He had severe injuries to his brain, chest, spine, abdomen, and limbs. Fractured ribs had punctured his lungs; catheters had to be placed between his ribs, into his chest cavity, so that suction could be applied to re-expand his collapsed lungs. A fractured spine threatened to paralyze him. His facial bones were broken, as was his right arm; he had at least ten fractures of his legs, including his left tibia (shin bone), which was exposed, protruding through the skin, and deformed. Excessive pressure was building from a blood clot on his swollen brain, a condition that can kill within minutes.

Alcides' condition was so precarious that moving him was risky, but he needed surgery, and he needed intensive care. We accomplished both by operating on him in his bed in the intensive care unit (ICU), including drilling a hole in his skull to relieve the pressure from his swelling brain, washing out the debris from his open tibia fracture and stabilizing it, and opening his abdomen to relieve the pressure that accumulated from the massive amounts of fluid and blood he required. Three operations, in bed, in the ICU! We pumped heated blood and fluid into him to warm his body temperature in the face of severe bleeding because his blood clotting system was failing. He continued losing blood, requiring more and more transfusions—a vicious cycle because the more blood we gave him, the more we diluted the clotting factors in his system that could have slowed the bleeding, and the more he bled. In the early hours we transfused him with more than twenty-five liters (six gallons) of blood products, some of which came back out of him, in the form of ongoing bleeding, as fast as we could administer it.

Alcides survived the night. Disbelief upon disbelief. This was truly uncharted territory for me and my team of dedicated surgeons, anesthesiologists, radiologists, nurses, and technicians. None of us had never seen survival in a situation like this and couldn't imagine Alcides would be an exception. Yet there he was in our ICU, comatose, but still alive. What now? A lot more work, many more operations to come. As he began to stabilize, there was time to ask questions and seek answers. If he was to survive, would his be a functional life, an enjoyable life, a meaningful life? At that point, there was no way to know for sure, so we kept working.

Through the month of December, he hung on. Unconscious and unresponsive, yet with normal vital signs, he remained attached to machines and monitors. He required more than twenty operations, orthopedic and others. How does the patient endure? With liberal administration of pain medication and sedatives—the so-called "medically induced coma." The answer to the big question still eluded us—we didn't know if he would ever awaken or what his brain function would be like if he did, but we had to prepare his broken body for the possibility that he might. That included trying to awaken him every day to see if his brain had started working again.

Alcides' wife was at his bedside constantly, lifting his hand to stroke her face and hair, speaking to him in hopes he could sense her presence. And then, on Christmas Day, he opened his eyes, reached for his wife, found a nurse's face instead, stroked it and said, "What did I do?" Later, his wife would tease him about stroking another woman's face. We were all astonished—an understatement—by his survival and his recovery of brain and speech function. As human interest stories go, there was none better. Ever. More amazement was to follow.

Through it all, Alcides showed determination and courage and, with the love of his wife and family, became the only person I have ever known to survive a fall of this magnitude. Unprecedented, in the purest form of the word. How did he survive? The surgeon-scientist in me knows he landed on his legs rather than his torso or head. He received excellent pre-hospital care and emergency care. Brilliant surgeons did brilliant operations, time and time again. His nursing care was vigilant, skilled, and compassionate. Importantly, he never developed a serious infection as a complication of his care.

But how was he still alive to make it to the hospital in the first place? That I do not know. Perhaps it was the hand of God, cupping him gently and lowering him to the pavement. What do you believe? And how to explain the survival of only one of the two brothers?

Alcides was hospitalized for about two months. Thereafter he underwent many months of grueling physical therapy and rehabilitation. He received psychotherapy as well to deal with his brother's death—he and his brother had been close. In 2014, seven years after his fall, a New York newspaper did a follow-up story on Alcides' progress. Now living in Arizona with his family, he told the paper the warm climate helps his bones feel better. He drives his children to school and works out in a gym. Not only is he able to walk normally, he does charity walks to benefit others.

If you are a believer in miracles, this would be one.

To read a contemporary account of the circumstances surrounding Alcides' injury, see:

http://www.nydailynews.com/news/e-side-scaffold-fall-horror-brothers-article-1.273404

To read a contemporary account of a press conference held at the family's request to discuss his recovery and prognosis, in which this essayist is quoted extensively, see:

http://www.nytimes.com/2008/01/04/nyregion/04fall.html?pagewanted=all&_r=0

To read the 2014 follow-up newspaper article on Alcides, see:

http://nypost.com/2014/01/05/window-washer-survived-47-story-plunge-now-walks-for-charity/

To read the 2003 medical report on the man who fell "only" 19 stories, see:

Lee BS, Eachempati SR, Bacchetta MD, Levine MR, Barie PS. Survival after a documented 19-story fall: A case report. *J Trauma*. 2003 Nov; 55: 869–872.

To read the 2009 medical report of Alcides' case, see:

Kepler CK, Nho SJ, Miller AN, Barie PS, Lyden JP. Orthopaedic injuries associated with fall from floor forty-seven. *J Orthop Trauma* 2009; 23: 154–158.

DATE OF EVENT: SEPTEMBER 2008

Decapitated

Richard Roberts, MD

Jordan was nine years old at the time of the devastating accident. He was in the backseat, buckled up, when a dump truck collided with the car his mom was driving. The force of the impact was so severe it literally tore Jordan's skull from his neck and pitched it forward. The medical term for this type of injury is an *atlanto-occipital dislocation*, also known as an internal decapitation. All of the soft tissues inside the neck that keep the head connected were destroyed and his head was dangling, unattached by anything except his skin and the most superficial neck tissues. His mom later said that when she looked into the backseat after the horrific collision, it looked like Jordan's head was just dangling in front of him. She didn't know how right she was.

I was the neurosurgeon (brain surgeon) who was in charge of Jordan's care. My first question upon his arrival to the hospital and after seeing the X-ray studies was, "Is he still alive?"

As soon as I evaluated him, I knew how severe his injuries were. His MRI test (a special type of imaging study) showed that all of the soft tissues under the skin of his neck were destroyed. Survival from this type of injury is less than 1 percent, and among those very few who survive, paralysis and brain damage are the rule. Although Jordan's spinal cord was, miraculously, not severed, I didn't know how badly it may have been traumatized. What

I did know was that his head and neck had to be immediately stabilized to prevent his spinal cord from further injury.

I put him into a *halo vest*, a carbon-fiber ring that is fixed to the skull with sharp pins, and then attached to a vest on his torso with rods to temporarily hold his head in a stable position. A torture device, to be sure, but still the best way to stabilize his neck. We then took him to the operating room where I attached a titanium plate to his skull and titanium rods and screws from the plate to his spinal column to keep his skull attached to his spine. After surgery, in the intensive care unit, we allowed ourselves to believe for the first time that he would likely survive, but we still had no way of knowing whether or not he'd be paralyzed, or have other brain or spinal damage from the injury. In the early hours and days it didn't look good. The left side of his body was weak, suggesting there had indeed been some stretching or bruising of the spinal nerves. And he wasn't speaking, raising the concern of brain damage.

But in the weeks following surgery, Jordan shocked all of us with his astounding recovery. With the help of intense physical therapy, he went from a wheelchair to a walker to walking on his own. His speech came back and the weakness on his left side resolved. When he left the hospital, three months after his accident and several days before Christmas, he did so on his own power. Incredibly, he returned to school after winter break. Because of the rods and screws attaching his skull to his spine, his neck movements will always be somewhat restricted, but otherwise he is neurologically back to normal.

This is the first case of internal decapitation I have ever seen survive. It's an injury that is almost always catastrophic, almost always fatal. Most patients never make it past the accident scene, dead on arrival to the emergency room. Of those who do survive, a nearly full recovery like Jordan's is virtually unheard of.

In media interviews when her son was discharged from the hospital, Jordan's mom called this the best Christmas miracle she could ever have imagined. I agree and, along with fine teams of caregivers—beginning at the accident scene, on to the emergency room and operating room, in the intensive care and transitional care units, and all the way through rehabilitation and hospital discharge—it was a privilege to have been a part of it.

When Lightning Struck

James K. Todd, MD

I t was July 1, the first day of my first clinical rotations as a third-year medical student, far too early for me to have decided what area of medicine I would ultimately like best. After all, I had never really taken care of a patient of any kind yet, and there was so much I didn't know.

This was my pediatrics rotation, and I was assigned to a typical county hospital with very limited resources, staffed by a few senior physicians, residents, and medical students like me from the large, state university medical school. It was a Saturday that began bright and sunny, but became cloudy with severe thunderstorms in the afternoon. I had just gotten oriented to the pediatrics ward when a call came from the emergency room that I should come immediately. A six-year-old girl had been playing in her backyard when lightning struck a metal clothesline and sparked down one of the poles, leaving little Fern breathless and without a heartbeat.

The firemen responded quickly and found her barely breathing and having violent seizures. As soon as she arrived at the emergency room, staff quickly inserted a breathing tube through her mouth into her trachea. They were using a self-inflating resuscitation bag connected to the tube, pumped by hand, to breathe for her.

"Here," said the senior resident handing me the bag, "you keep her going while we see to some other emergencies." The doctors had heavily sedated her to slow her seizures, which had the unfortunate side effect of stopping her breathing altogether. It was all they could do under the circumstances. I sat there for what seemed like hours watching every heartbeat on the monitor. If I slowed down my hand-pumping of the bag, her heart rate would begin to slow as well, indicating she wasn't getting enough oxygen. This tube and bag were the only things keeping her alive.

By evening, it was obvious we had to make other arrangements for Fern's care. We didn't have a pediatric intensive care unit, she couldn't stay in the emergency room because of lack of space, and we certainly didn't have the staff to keep breathing for her by hand-pumping the bag.

"Do you know how to run a ventilator (mechanical breathing machine)?" asked the pediatrics resident in charge of the nursery.

I had no idea—this was my first day wearing my white coat as a medical student in a hospital! This hospital had just two newborn baby breathing machines that were used for small premature infants; one was available.

"I don't know if it will work for someone this big, but it's all we've got," he said.

Still hand-bagging her, I moved Fern to a room across from the pediatric nursing station. We hooked her up to the newborn breathing machine that was run off a pressurized oxygen line. There were only a few dials that allowed adjustments so we fine-tuned it the same way I had learned how to adjust a sail as I headed the boat close into the wind—pull the tiller in a bit while tightening up on the main sheet. Sailing was all a matter of trial and error, with constant attention to the wind indicators and the speed and direction of the boat. In trying to adjust the dials on this breathing machine, I watched her chest rise and fall with each pressurized burst of the machine, and made sure that her heart rate didn't drop.

"Good work," the resident said. "Don't go anywhere for the rest of the weekend. You are all she's got. There's no one else who knows how to run this machine."

God help us, I thought, *we're in big trouble if* I'm *the knowledgeable one.*

The nurses brought a bed in for me, but I don't remember having slept a bit the next two days. It was July 4th, and we had tried several times to wean her off the sedation that was controlling her seizures and suppressing her breathing, but every time she would start having seizures again. Her devoted and grieving parents, who had been continuously at the bedside with me, were losing hope and so was I. It seemed like we weren't making any progress. Fostered by exhaustion and self-doubt, questions raced through my mind. *Should we give up? Is this what a career in medicine is going to be like?*

The nurses insisted I go home for some much-needed rest. By then, the ward resident and another student had learned how to keep the breathing machine going, but we were all concerned that her brain had been too badly damaged from lack of adequate oxygen and seizures. I was exhausted, both emotionally and physically, even more the former because of the realization that Fern's life had been solely in my inexperienced hands for almost three days and yet her condition remained grave.

I slept through Independence Day and have no recollection of any fireworks; they could have exploded right next to me and I doubt that I would have noticed. The next morning, I hurried back to the hospital, my own heart racing with the fear that Fern had not made it. As I walked down the hallway, I saw several of the nurses looking excitedly toward me. They disappeared and then, probably with their coaxing, little Fern came around the corner walking unsteadily toward me. Miraculously, while I had slept, her seizures had stopped and she had been quickly weaned off the ventilator.

"Thank you, Dr. Todd," she said as I dropped to one knee to hold her with tears of joy in my eyes. I wasn't even close to being a doctor yet, but at that moment, even though this was only my first clinical experience, I knew I was destined to be a pediatrician. I had witnessed the resiliency of young life, its ability to heal and to adjust to adversity. Fern's parents later told me the only difference they saw in their little girl after her recovery was that she had previously been right-handed. They presented me with a picture their now perfectly normal daughter had drawn for me, now with her left hand. A few circuits may have been scrambled by the lightning, but not her essential spirit. Having endured for agonizing days the ordeal of helplessly watching their daughter having seizures and unable to breathe for herself, they were so thankful—and so was I.

There would be many times in the years that followed, as I cared for other desperately ill children in the intensive care unit, that I would remember Fern. She had taught me that, beyond the limits of my medical knowledge and skill, there is also always the power of hope.

DATE OF EVENT: 2005

Shrapnel—
I Knew He Had Lost His Eye

Robert J. Buys

Before I ever met Joe, I knew he had lost his eye.

It was all there in the black-and-white X-ray image of his eye sockets—a large piece of metal lodged in the back of the eye. This is called an *intraocular foreign body* (IOFB), meaning an object within the eye that shouldn't be there. Joe's story was a common one for this type of incident—and so typically frustrating. A piece of metal had exploded off an axe during log-splitting. He was not actually using the axe—he was several feet away. As the metal projectile raced through the air it heated up and probably became sterile from the friction. That is where the good news for Joe ended. It is not unusual for flying projectiles to hit the one soft spot on the face—the eye—as it did with Joe. Or maybe when an object hits elsewhere on the bonier parts of the face, victims don't require medical attention as often. Regardless, when a flying projectile is headed in the direction of the eye, the eye seems to lock in on the incoming missile so, invariably, the vital structures in the center of the eye, the center of visual focus, are hit. Structures crucial for vision, like the optic nerve, which transmits visual images to our brain, or the macula, which is the structure responsible for our main central vision and the source of our greatest visual acuity, are damaged. The bigger the IOFB the greater the chances are that the damage will be catastrophic. And this was a big one.

Joe was just a kid—floppy blond hair, smooth skin, round face, full of the innocence toward life that all twelve-year-olds seem to have. At this age, he'd yet to hit the really big milestones that would mark his passage from childhood to adulthood: getting a driver's license, senior prom, graduation, attending college. I was certain this accident would affect all those events in ways we couldn't predict just yet. For now, all I could see was a kid facing the first truly big crisis of his life.

As I met the family I tried to assess his home situation. Would he have the support needed to get through this? The parents were on the verge of tears, very concerned, and full of love and compassion. They were older folks who, as it turned out, were not his parents but his grandparents. There was something in the way the grandfather rubbed his hands, dropped his head, could barely speak. It was not just love and concern—guilt. He had been the one using the axe and he blamed himself.

My physical examination of Joe's eye revealed the path the piece of metal had taken—an entry site in the cornea, the clear surface structure of the eye. From there it traversed the fluid-filled front chamber without causing any bleeding, and then into the iris (the pupil). His lens was clear, but that can be falsely reassuring—often cataracts will form and cloud the lens sometime after the trauma. The pressure within the eye was low, as would be expected with an open wound. My view to the back of the eye was blocked by blood within the vitreous, the jelly-like substance that fills the back chamber of the eye. His visual acuity was extremely poor—he could only see my hand moving in front of his face.

It was close to midnight when the surgery began. What would be required would be a three-stage procedure. First, I would have to repair the wound to the cornea. Then, an operation called a *pars plana vitrectomy*. The *pars plana* is a structure in the eye that provides access to the back chamber of the eye; vitrectomy means the removal of the gelatinous fluid in that chamber. In this case, the procedure would remove the blood that had accumulated in that back chamber. Finally, I would have to make a large incision to get the IOFB out of the eye. In young patients the vitreous is well formed and sticks to the retina at the back of the eye. This presents a challenge to the surgeon, particularly in the early stages of trauma. The retina is the vital structure in our eyes that processes light—without the retina, or with a severely damaged retina, a patient will be blind.

I cleared the blood and looked around for the piece of metal. I carefully examined where it had hit the retina—on the nasal side, causing no damage to the optic nerve or macula that I could see. Remarkable. But I could not find the metal! Often the IOFB bounces off the retina and can lodge away from the impact site. I returned to the impact site and carefully examined it. I could feel the tip of the metal beneath the retina. The IOFB had travelled from the cornea, clear through the vitreous and the retina, and was now lodged in the sclera behind the eye—a through-and-through wound called a double perforation. I could not budge it from its final resting spot, despite trying with magnets and probes. I had no choice but to leave it there and live to fight another day. I closed the incision in the eye and removed the surgical drapes on the patient's face, revealing, to my horror, the most unusual post-operative situation I have ever seen.

Incredibly, the eyeball was bulging out of the socket as far as humanly possible. He looked like a something from a sci-fi movie. I could not relieve the massive swelling, could not even close the lids over the eye. The operating room went silent and my worst nightmare was literally staring me in the face. It was late at night, I was exhausted, and the fate of Joe's eye was hanging in the balance. And I had no idea what to do. I covered the eye with ointment, put a patch on, and wondered what had happened. Had he bled into the eye socket as I probed for the IOFB? I faced the grandparents and wondered how I was going to possibly take the patch off the next day.

I knew then he had lost his eye.

The next morning, only five hours after the surgery, I removed the patch, prepared for what I thought would be an ugly sight. I could not believe what I saw—the eye was back to normal and his vision was actually pretty good! I could see to the very back of the eye, and the retina was attached. My only explanation was that as I cleared the gelatinous fluid from the impact site, or perhaps during my attempts to get at the piece of metal, the exit wound became open and the fluid I was infusing during the procedure left the eye and went to the eye socket. This had created the bulging and now that excess fluid had been reabsorbed. I was counting my lucky stars—a miracle had saved the eye—and Joe's vision was improving!

But it was not to be.

Within a week everything had changed; the retina had now completely detached from the back of eye. Stiff folds of the retina emanated from the impact site. Joe's vision was back to hand motions only. Again my heart sank; I had been down this road many times before. In children, even if you can get the retina attached initially, there is a high probability that it will detach again due to a scarring process known as *proliferative vitreoretinopathy*. And if the detached retina wasn't bad enough, with the severe trauma and two operations, I considered cataract formation inevitable.

I knew then he had lost his eye.

Back to the operating room. I removed any stickiness left from the gelatinous vitreous fluid, freed the delicate retina from the impact site, and removed the blood that had accumulated under the retina. I then drained the rest of the fluid under the retina and filled the eye with air. Next, I exchanged the air with a longer-lasting gas that would hold the retina in place while it healed. Joe would have to keep his head down for weeks. A great excuse to play video games all day long.

That great family support I had seen that first night played a key role. When I first met Joe he seemed terrified—but as I got to know him I realized he was composed, determined, and confident of success. Miraculously, the eye healed, the retina never detached again, the lens remained clear without cataracts, and his vision became a near-perfect 20/25.

Somehow a large metal shard tore through his eye, completely missing the vital and irreplaceable optic nerve and macula. The shard eventually detached the retina, but Joe dodged every expected complication and ended up with a completely unexpected and fantastic result.

Joe grew up to be great young man, went to high school, and attended leadership camps with my enthusiastic letters of recommendation. The metal remains lodged behind his eye to this day.

I know now I had been wrong all along.

EDITOR'S NOTE: The miracles didn't stop with this boy's recovery. The grateful family became committed to helping save others' vision, as well; their generosity is evidenced in another essay in this book, "The Thin Line Between Miracle and Tragedy."

DATE OF EVENT: LABOR DAY 2011

Shredded

Valerie Pruitt, MD

I t was Labor Day weekend and a perfect day for enjoying the lakes of the Midwest. At the time, BobbieJo was a ten-year-old girl riding on a pontoon boat with her sister, dad, and uncle. Wearing her life vest, she was watching the water at the front of the boat when the boat decelerated and she was thrown overboard. She went under the boat and was ensnared in the boat propeller. Reacting quickly, her father immediately shut off the engine and raised the propeller, but his little girl was still submerged and he knew every second counted. He got his knife and cut her clothing loose from the propeller blades and dragged her back into the boat. They called 911 from the boat, and then sped to the nearest dock where they met the ambulance. She was transported to a local hospital where she was put on a breathing machine, because of a significant lung injury, and given a blood transfusion. Arrangements were then made to urgently airlift her to our facility, the nearest one with trauma care.

I was the trauma surgeon on call that evening and quickly examined her in the trauma bay of the emergency room. Her injuries were devastating. She was literally shredded, with multiple deep cuts from the propeller on her chest, chin, arm and leg. The worst slices were on her chest, where eight ribs were cut in half and her lung was protruding out of her chest. Her lung had collapsed, and we detected bleeding in her liver and a small cut on her diaphragm (the breathing muscle between the chest and the abdomen). It was evident that if she was to have any chance at all, she needed to go to the operating room immediately. In this first of what would ultimately be many surgeries, I put her lung back into her chest and repaired her ribs. I determined her liver and diaphragm would heal on their own and not require repair. I cleansed the cuts and tears as carefully as I could, but I remained very concerned that the potential for infection from the dirty lake water and propeller blades was very high.

After coming out of the operating room, I went to update her family, who had all arrived by that time. Her mother had not been on the boat but had been summoned from a leisurely Saturday to get to the hospital. She was overwhelmed with worry and fear for her daughter's life. Her father was still shaking from the tragic events of the accident. I carefully, and as gently as I could, explained BobbieJo's many injuries, what I had done in the operating room, and the upcoming need for many more surgeries. I tried to realistically assess for them BobbieJo's chances for survival and recovery. The picture was not rosy, no matter how much I tried to leave them with hope.

I am a general trauma surgeon trained to provide acute and urgent care for children and adults, but the hospital we were in was not a pediatric hospital. We were in a smaller town than where this child and her family lived, and they were understandably concerned about our experience in situations like this and the quality of care we could provide. The family asked to have the child moved to a different hospital and to the care of a specialized pediatric surgeon who might be more experienced in the types of ongoing surgery BobbieJo would undoubtedly need. Frankly, there aren't many cases like this in anyone's experience, but I knew that wouldn't reassure the family.

After the exhausting surgery and the immense tension surrounding saving this little girl's life, my emotions were mixed that night. I certainly understood BobbieJo's parents' desire to have her in the best possible care setting and in the best possible hands. I also understood their wanting to be closer to home—our facility was more than a three-hour drive from where they lived. But I was also deeply saddened after pouring out every drop of energy, knowledge, and skill to save this child's life, only to feel as if it hadn't been enough to earn the family's confidence for her future care. It was late in the evening so we stabilized BobbieJo for the night with plans to transfer her in the morning to a center closer to their home.

BobbieJo spent the night in our intensive care unit, with me checking on her frequently. There were no major crises that night. The next morning, the family had changed their mind and asked me to continue caring for their child in our facility. I felt gratified, but also somewhat apprehensive about the new and even greater responsibility of trying to bring this child back from the brink all the way to normal. She was far from normal that morning, and I wasn't certain she ever would be again. Now that would be on my shoulders; I felt personally and completely responsible for whatever outcome she might have.

Over the next nine days I performed five additional major surgeries on BobbieJo and countless wound cleanings. And I prayed, and I cried. I have a daughter this same age and very much felt the agony this family was in. The family's community rallied behind them, and their church held fundraisers in their hometown to help with the family's expenses. Thankfully, after an extended time in the hospital and the care of a wonderful team of physicians, nurses, and therapists, she had a truly remarkable recovery. The family called it a miracle, and I have to agree. Every one of BobbieJo's injuries healed without complications and none of her multiple and extensive wounds ever became infected. BobbieJo's family spent weeks in our small community, away from home, before she was ready for discharge; her mother never left her side.

During that time and on our journey together, her family and I developed a mutual respect, admiration, and friendship. I was proud of the commitment and faith her family showed, and of the courage and spirit BobbieJo found deep inside her to get through this ordeal.

We went from a day of horror to a time of relief and gratitude.

DATE OF EVENT: 1984

Kidnapped: The Story of Two Three-Year-Olds

Richard D. Krugman, MD

The lead story on the evening news was about a missing three-year-old. She and her four-year-old brother had been playing in their front yard on a warm August day when a car pulled up, the side door opened, she took off her underpants, and got into the car. Her brother raced inside their home to get their parents, but by the time they all got back outside, the car and the little girl were gone. The police were called and for the next two days, they, her parents, and the community frantically searched for her.

Two days later, the morning television shows were interrupted with breaking news. The girl had been found alive! Two birdwatchers walking in the foothills west of town—twenty miles from the front yard—heard what sounded like a child crying nearby. They followed the sound to an outhouse in a campground and opened the door. Down at the bottom of the outhouse, in the waste well, a little girl was crouched in a corner, shivering. Miraculously, this particular outhouse had a leak and there was no fluid in the well. Had it not leaked, she surely would have drowned.

"What are you doing there?" one rescuer asked.

"I live here," the dazed and confused little girl said. "It's my home."

The girl was taken by helicopter to a local general hospital trauma center. TV cameras captured her parents racing into the hospital to be reunited with their daughter. Within a half hour after her arrival, the physicians told dozens of gathered reporters that "She was dehydrated, but going to be fine," and "She had not been sexually abused."

At the time, I was director of a center for the prevention of child abuse, where we were anxiously following the story on television with the rest of the city. We were grateful and relieved she was found alive, but skeptical about the last statement made by the doctors. In our experience, the kidnapping of three-year-old girls was often motivated by sexual abuse.

I, along with our child abuse prevention center, became involved in this case a week later. The police department investigating the matter wanted to show a videotape they had made of a lineup. The tape showed the girl, sitting in her mother's lap, watching as six men were asked, one by one, to step forward and say: "Take off your pants and get into the car."

When the fourth man finished saying those words, the girl blurted out: "Mommy! That's him! That's the bad man who put me in the hole."

The question the police detective had for us was, "Is her statement reliable?" The child psychiatrist and the attorney at our center agreed that it was reliable, but it would not be admissible in court. However, they believed a videotaped interview under the right circumstances might be.

On Saturday morning of Labor Day weekend we did a ninety-minute "play interview" with the three-year-old. I ran the video camera as our child psychiatrist skillfully asked her about her experience from the time she got into the car until she was found. She played out the events with toys, demonstrating everything she could remember, including her unmistakable sexual abuse. Months later, when the individual who had kidnapped her confessed as part of a plea bargain, his confession could have been the subtitles to her videotaped interview. The accuracy of the little girl's videotaped testimony was perfect.

Our center treated the little girl for the next year. The following fall, she walked into our waiting area where her therapist and I were expecting her, and—now a self-confident four-year-old—she said, pointing to the psychiatrist, "You are my talking doctor! He (pointing to me) is my real doctor. I am done talking!" I was her pediatrician for the next three years.

Twelve years later, I was dean of the school of medicine. My secretary buzzed me and said that there was someone on the phone who wanted to talk with me; did I have a minute? It was my former patient, now eighteen and doing a term paper on child abuse. She wondered if she could interview me, and if so, would the next day at 4:00 work? My calendar said I had an important meeting at that time, but I said, "Absolutely."

She came in the next afternoon and had nineteen questions for me. It took twenty-five minutes to answer them. After a pause, she looked at me and said: "My mom tells me that you and the psychiatrist saved my life. I just wanted to say thank you." It was an amazing moment in my career—and, even though it was nearly midnight in England where her former "talking doctor" lived, we called him on the phone, woke him up, and he and our former patient had a wonderful conversation. He visited with her and her parents the following year when he came to town for a conference on child abuse.

Now, more than thirty years after her kidnapping and attempted murder, this little girl is a happily married mother of three. She has her master's degree in counseling and a successful practice helping others. Many believe that if you were abused as a child, you will be an abuser. That turns out to not be true. More than two-thirds of abused children never repeat the cycle and many, like this remarkable three-year-old, do very, very well.

However, in our experience, it is true that all abusers have themselves been abused in childhood. Our center psychiatrist interviewed the man who kidnapped our patient while he served his sentence in our state prison. He denied being abused, but when he described his childhood and what his brothers did to him, it was almost certain he was abused. Neighbors who lived on the same cul-de-sac he lived on told us that they recall him wandering from yard to yard as a little three-year-old, seemingly "lost" or looking to get away from his house. These former neighbors told me they wished they knew then what they know now about child abuse and neglect so they could have reported the family in hopes of protecting the child.

The life trajectories of these two abused three-year-olds, who grew up a generation apart in our community and crossed paths one day in August, took them in very different directions. One went to prison, the other to a productive life helping others. One was lost to the vicious cycle of child abuse, the other miraculously saved by an unlikely convergence of Good Samaritans walking near a leaking outhouse.

These three-year-olds remind us of the fragility of childhood, and our collective obligation to work toward building a society that can better protect children from harm.

6

Mysterious Presence

We are trained to be keen observers in delivering care to our patients and, when they are critically ill, our five senses go on high alert. Subtle or dramatic changes in a patient's condition alert us to the possible need to take action. A shift in a patient's mood may indicate an important emotional or psychological need. The concerns of our patients' families also rise to prominent places in our consciousness, as does the setting in which we find our patients—the clinic or hospital room, the blinking lights and beeping monitors.

Yet there are times when our five senses may not be enough. Times when something beyond our awareness may be even more important in coming to grips with unfolding events.

DATE OF EVENT: 1996

The Boy Who Saw Heaven

Joanne Hilden, MD

The mother of a five-year-old boy suffering a relapse of *neuroblastoma*, a very serious type of childhood cancer, was in clinic with her son to discuss options, none of them very good. His tumor was not responding to the latest round of chemotherapy, which included medicines with more serious side effects, given only when more standard treatment doesn't work. He was a quiet child, her only child. His grandmother sometimes came to clinic with them, but not this time.

The tumor had come back after multiple rounds of chemotherapy, and the child was noticeably weak. He had been through many lengthy and difficult experiences with his disease and his therapy, including several long hospitalizations with fever and severe blood infections. As his oncologist (cancer doctor), I tried to counsel his mother that since the tumor kept coming back on chemotherapy, she should consider the use of a gentler form of chemotherapy intended to slow the growth of the tumor, rather than still hoping for a remission or cure using high-dose chemotherapy. I told them that with the high-dose approach, we would again be harming the boy's immune system and making him susceptible to serious infections as he had been before. The gentler approach, I explained, might allow them to enjoy some time out of the hospital before he died.

The mother's desire was for continued aggressive treatment, trying everything we could to achieve remission or cure and, following her wishes, that is what we did. During the period that followed this new round of aggressive treatment, the little boy was again hospitalized with fever due to extremely low blood counts and infections. He was bedridden with very little energy and did not talk much, requiring high doses of morphine for pain.

As his care team, we became accustomed to this child sleeping most of the day and being in pain when he was awake. The Child Life team at the hospital was not able to get him to play during those awake periods. We visited him many times during the day. His blood cultures grew bacteria again, requiring IV antibiotics. Any discussion of getting him home into a hospice-type environment where we could make him more comfortable was met with instant resistance by the family who wanted to try everything possible to fight the cancer. So the hospital became his new home in this end stage of his life.

It was a Friday and we saw him at the end of morning rounds. The room was somber, with his family there in deep distress and sadness due to the child's obvious deterioration and failure, again, to respond to treatment. He was lying very still, breathing quietly. His room was near the nurses' desk, so the sounds of a busy hospital were present.

Then suddenly, this frail and previously motionless child sat up in bed. He sat straight up, and looked right past us all. His blank expression turned slowly into one of absolute joy. It was a slowly dawning, big wonderful smile; his eyes especially seemed peaceful and happy. His smile grew bigger and bigger, with his eyes still looking right past us.

Some sort of instinct filled me. I took his hand and put it in his mother's hand, and said, "Mommy's here."

As I and the three other caregivers in the room witnessed this little boy's sudden, mesmerized behavior, we felt as if we were in a state of suspended animation. No one wanted to do or say anything to interrupt the moment. To this day, I cannot remember how long his fixated glow lasted, but the next thing he did was simply lie down. He then took his last breath, his hand intertwined with his mother's.

Every last one of us believes we watched our little friend see heaven that morning.

The Man All Dressed in White

Kathleen Farrell, MD

I was a second-year resident at a large Midwest children's hospital on call overnight in the pediatric intensive care unit. A two-year-old near-drowning patient was admitted with pneumonia due to inhaled pool water, resulting in severe respiratory failure. The chest X-ray showed a complete "white out," meaning all the air spaces were completely filled by fluid.

After stabilizing the patient with a breathing tube, mechanical ventilator (breathing machine), sedation, oxygen, and intravenous fluids, I and the medical student working with me that evening sat down with the family to learn what had happened. The little boy had toddled into the deep end of the swimming pool at a family reunion that evening where none of the family members knew how to swim. The medical student asked who lifted the toddler from the pool and the five-year-old cousin proudly piped up, "I did!"

Indeed, the uncle confirmed he saw her bring the toddler to the surface in the shallow end of the pool and he, the uncle, then immediately started CPR (cardiopulmonary resuscitation). Our medical student asked the five-year-old, "What made you go get your cousin in the bottom of the pool when you don't know how to swim yourself?"

She answered excitedly, "That's easy, the man all dressed in white told me to."

We were stunned by her answer. Our astonishment continued through the evening as we watched how quickly the patient improved after arriving entirely nonresponsive and in severe respiratory distress. Overnight, our patient easily weaned off the oxygen and ventilator, and was up playing in bed, talking, entirely back to normal. The chest X-ray was now also normal, no traces of fluid. *Impossible!*

That morning on rounds, our medical student described to the team what the cousin had stated and how amazed we were with the toddler's seemingly miraculous improvement. At the end of the presentation our supervising attending physician said, "Great, he can transfer out of intensive care to the floor. Let's make sure the family gets swim lessons, so next time we don't have to rely on the angels to save him."

I don't know if our supervisor's guardian angels comment was sincere or sarcastic, but to this day I don't have a better explanation for what happened at the pool or in its aftermath.

DATE OF EVENT: SPRING 2001

A Sea of Blood

Matthew A. Metz, MD

I was a second-year surgery resident, near the bottom of the totem pole in the highly hierarchical world of surgery. I was "scrubbed in" for an abdominal procedure with a team of outstanding surgeons at a world-class medical center in upstate New York. My role was largely to watch and learn. If I was fortunate, I might be asked to hold the "retractor" tool, or perhaps the surgeon in charge would let me help with closing the surgical skin wound after the important work inside the abdomen was finished.

This was to have been a fairly routine procedure to remove a sarcoma tumor in the groin from an otherwise healthy sixty-year-old woman, but once the head surgeon began the procedure, everything went quickly wrong.

As he began to remove the mass, bleeding began. The tumor had grown into the femoral vein, the major vein in the groin, and the attempt to remove the tumor tore the vein, filling the surgical field of view with a sea of blood. To make matters worse, the vein had withdrawn up into the abdomen when the tumor mass was cut away, and the uncontrolled bleeding now filled the entire abdomen.

Frantically, the surgeon tried to find and stem the source of bleeding. But as quickly as the team suctioned the blood away, more blood filled the void. The surgeon reached in with his gloved hand, trying to grip the bleeding vessel, or vessels, to "tourniquet" the gusher. Nothing. He wasn't able to find the "bleeder" with any of his tools or with his hands.

I was horrified by what I was seeing, and certain, as everyone else around the operating table was, that this was going to be a tragedy for this patient and for all of us. In what must have been a burst of adrenaline and irrational panic, I heard myself saying, "Can I try?" *Can I try? What was I thinking?* Who was I to even imagine I could do something the entire senior team in the room was unable to do? As soon as the words left my mouth, I knew I had probably committed a career-ending blunder—I'd be politely asked to reconsider my decision to be a surgeon, or perhaps offered a residency as a pathologist where the patients were already dead.

It was a sign of the desperation in the room, the reconciliation everyone felt with the inevitable catastrophe playing out in front of them, that the chief surgeon looked at me with a smirk and said, "Sure, Metz, here you go," and handed me the tool he was using, a *vascular needle driver*, a special kind of forceps for holding a needle and a suture (surgical thread) to stitch up a hole in a blood vessel. A great device if you can see the blood vessel and find the hole—neither of which was possible in this case.

What happened next remains a blur after all these years. I grabbed the needle driver and the attached needle and suture and plunged my hand blindly into the sea of blood in the abdominal cavity. Somehow, the needle and suture ended up precisely where the hole in the vein was, and I was quickly able to draw the two sides of the tear together. To the audible awe and amazement of everyone in the room, the bleeding stopped. At that moment, the adrenaline receded from my body almost instantly, and my knees went weak. I leaned against the table, accepting the stunned congratulations from the others surrounding it. The patient not only survived the surgery, but went on to a full recovery.

I would tell my colleagues afterward that I didn't deserve their congratulations. I have no idea what happened in that woman's abdomen that morning, but I do know this: it wasn't me guiding my hand to that blood vessel.

DATE OF EVENT: SPRING 1989

The Miracle Within Us

David Slamowitz, MD

I have always been interested in the unseen forces that shape our world and impact our health. Even as a child I recall being fascinated by such things as magic, sorcery, science, martial arts, meditation, and hypnosis. I tried to read whatever I could find on my subjects of interest. However, when it came to hypnosis, the available reading material in my local library was quite minimal. Most of the literature would describe the characteristics of being in a hypnotic trance without truly explaining the process of how to attain the state itself.

It wasn't until many years later that I was finally able to witness the power of hypnosis over the mind-body connection firsthand. I had just completed my second year of medical school and was about to begin my clinical rotations. This involved four- to eight-week stints working with supervising physicians in each of the major fields of medicine. Psychiatry was my first clinical rotation. As part of my training, I was fortunate to be able to attend a six-week hypnosis course usually offered only to the psychiatry residents, young physicians who already finished medical school and were now specializing. During the course I learned some of the theory behind hypnosis as well as the practical steps needed to place someone into a hypnotic trance. The instructor spent time guiding me, along with the rest of the group, through the experience of a hypnotic induction, which leads one into the early phase of a hypnotic trance state. I found the course quite interesting intellectually, but could not say that I actually experienced any kind of altered state of consciousness or hypnotic trance. By the end of the course, I was somewhat skeptical about hypnosis as a therapeutic tool and considered the so-called hypnotic trance an interesting parlor trick—if it was actually a real entity at all.

I finished my psychiatry rotation and moved on to my next clinical experience, obstetrics and gynecology. On the first day, as I was just getting my bearings, I was told to visit a patient who had just undergone surgery for an *ectopic pregnancy*. An ectopic pregnancy occurs when the fetus begins growing in the fallopian tube rather than in the uterus. Those pregnancies cannot continue to term and surgery is typically required to remove the fetus before it ruptures the fallopian tube, which can be very dangerous. Both the ectopic pregnancy and the surgery to treat it are very painful. When I entered the patient's room, I found a twenty-something-year-old thin woman, moaning in pain, with no other healthcare staff in sight. At that moment, I certainly could have left the room in search of a nurse and pain medication for this young woman. However, a different spirit took hold. Without much thought, I asked her permission to attempt a hypnotic induction that I had recently learned from the hypnosis course to see if I could ease her pain. If it didn't work, I would immediately seek out some pain medication for her. She agreed to let me begin.

"Close your eyes and listen to what I am going to tell you," I told her. She did as she was asked, though she continued to moan in pain. I then worked through the induction steps as I had been taught. Surprisingly, the first thing I noticed was that her moaning stopped and she became quiet and still as her eyes remained closed. *Did she fall asleep?* That's when it started getting interesting. I moved on to the *deepening phase*, which follows the trance induction. I suggested to her that as her hand started to become lighter and lighter, her pain would begin to decrease. Well, to my utter amazement, her left hand began slowly lifting off the bed as if being pulled from above by a string. Not only that, once her hand attained a height of about six inches, it became stationary and perfectly still, remaining suspended in midair above the bed. I stood there almost in disbelief. *Wow! Maybe there really is something to this hypnosis!* I then suggested to her that her hand would start to become heavier and heavier, and as this happened her pain would continue to become less and less. Her hand slowly descended and once again rested lightly on the bed. Finally, I continued on to the *alerting phase* of the hypnosis session, transitioning her back to full consciousness. During this phase, I suggested to her that when she opened her eyes she would be fully awake and alert but would feel no pain. As she opened her eyes, the first words out of her mouth were, "Doc, I don't feel any pain!" And from the look of relief on her face, I truly believed she did not!

The experience of that special moment solidified my appreciation for the power of the mind and its ability to profoundly affect the body's physiology. Hypnosis is not a miracle, in the traditional sense. Neither, for that matter, is acupuncture, meditation, biofeedback, or relaxation therapy a miracle in the traditional sense. Unless, of course, you're the patient whose pain, stress, insomnia, anxiety, or panoply of other physical and mental health conditions has been relieved by mobilizing the power of the mind-body connection. These therapeutic tools are not like the magic and sorcery that so fascinated me as a child—the medical and scientific literature are filled with peer-reviewed studies (research published only after rigorous review by experts in the field) showing the benefits of each of these "alternative" therapies.

As a physician, what I believe is "miraculous" is the power within each of us to affect our health and our healing. Prescribing medicine is easy. Too easy.

Empowering our patients to harness the power of their mind-body connection may be more difficult, more time-consuming, and less remunerative—but in some ways may be even more rewarding. That's why physicians should endeavor to practice more of this type of health care, or at least be open to it, when solid evidence exists for its utility.

As a postscript, I went on to receive additional training in hypnosis, and a little over ten years after my patient raised and lowered her hand to relieve her pain, I began successfully using hypnosis as a therapeutic tool to treat insomnia. Now, many years later, I continue to use hypnosis regularly in my sleep medicine practice.

To ignore the power of the mind-body connection and to leave it untapped is to ignore the miracle within us.

DATE OF EVENT: LATE 1990s

Witnessing the Unknown

Meredith Belber, MD

I t was early in my career and I was caring for Lois, a woman in her late eighties with a serious heart condition, in the critical care unit. Her aortic valve was not functioning effectively, a potentially life-threatening condition not uncommon for someone her age. In an attempt to avoid open heart surgery, Lois underwent a less invasive procedure to repair the valve in hopes of providing her a few extra months of life to spend with her family.

The procedure was successful. A few days later while making my daily visit, I witnessed something I have never previously seen. I was standing next to her hospital bed, on her left, when she suddenly turned toward the door on the right and began talking to someone. She was engaged in this conversation for several minutes, speaking calmly, rationally, but with frustration. At first I thought she may be talking to someone out of my line of sight, but soon realized there was nobody there. Obviously, I only heard her end of the conversation, which consisted of her telling this person that she wanted to go. Lois said she was ready. She then became upset and asked why it wasn't time. Lois turned back to me and I asked to whom she had been speaking. She said, sounding surprised that I didn't know, "My husband." Her husband had died many years earlier. Instead of being frightened or unnerved, I remember feeling relieved. I wasn't the only one watching over Lois, responsible for the outcome of her life.

Several months later I saw Lois in my office for a follow-up visit. She told me that since the hospitalization, her husband had been visiting her regularly in her sleep and told her she could now join him. Lois died two weeks later.

Recently, I related this episode to a physician friend, who said his 101-year-old grandfather had a similar experience near death. After days of lying in a hospital bed with barely enough strength to move, drifting in and out of consciousness, his grandfather suddenly and vigorously lifted both arms straight up in the air. He began waving his arms, pointing, and repeating the phrase, "All the people, all the people," seeing what no one else in the room could see. This was disturbing and confusing to those watching it occur. The hospital chaplain happened to be one of those in the room at the time. When asked what had just happened, the chaplain said, "It's hard to ever know for sure, but we see this sometimes as patients are near death. They see things we don't." My friend's grandfather had no further episodes like that before his death several weeks later.

As a doctor, it always amazes me how much connection exists between this world and somewhere else. A dying patient's desire to spare the pain of those they love who will be left behind often seems to impact the outcome of events. Sometimes, when patients are near death, they seem to have some control over when the actual end occurs—perhaps making it quick to minimize the pain of those watching in agony, or lingering for a few hours longer to give traveling family members time to arrive from out of town and say their good-byes.

Sometimes I wonder if, as physicians, we do too much to interfere with these patients' transitions. There are times, I think, where we should just step back and let the patient decide how and when events should happen. It seems that's just what Lois did.

No matter what someone's religious beliefs may be, there is, without question in my mind, something greater that controls our lives, which the most intelligent physicians and modern science cannot touch. To me, that is more than just mysterious. It's "miraculous," and makes me feel honored and proud to be a part of something so special, being able to witness and acknowledge the unknown.

7

Global Miracles

In developed countries like the United States, where most of the events in this book take place, the miracles we witness as physicians typically involve individual patients. Yet in the developing world, where the needs of overwhelming numbers of people with devastating diseases are so great, the most effective type of health care is often that administered by global and public health providers who treat entire populations.

Two of the essays in this chapter are written by global health physicians describing miraculous encounters in their work that changed their lives, their careers, and their perspectives on health care in developing nations. The other essay is from a public health doctor fighting in the trenches of the AIDS war in Africa, where finding a way to sustain therapy for the neediest patients can require a miracle.

The Miracle
of a Single Sentence

Frank O. Richards Jr., MD

ONCE I WAS YOUNG AND SO UNSURE
I'D TRY ANY ILL TO FIND THE CURE
AN OLD MAN TOLD ME
TRYIN' TO SCOLD ME
"WHOA, SON, DON'T WADE TOO DEEP IN BITTER CREEK"

—The Eagles, *Desperado* album, 1973

I am a public health doctor, which means that my "patients" are entire communities and populations rather than individuals. Yet there was this poor old man living in the middle of nowhere who had one of the most significant and lasting impacts on my career and on my view of medicine. I think of him often, and I can see him as if it were yesterday. He helped me, scolded me, and also—perhaps—warned me about what I was wading into.

The setting was Guatemala in 1988. I was there as part of the public health team hoping to eradicate a parasite disease called "river blindness" or, more technically, *onchocerciasis*. Onchocerciasis is a leading cause of infection-related blindness in the world. The worm that causes it (*Onchocerca volvulus*) is transmitted by bites of certain black flies, and at that time the disease was rampant in Guatemala. In fact, the country was the most affected in Latin America, and the area where I was working was the most affected area in

Guatemala. Today, thanks to public and private health sector collaboration, Guatemala (and Latin America) is 95 percent of the way to reaching elimination of river blindness. That has been an important part of my life's work. . . . But I'm getting ahead of myself.

"Once I was young and so unsure
I'd try any ill to find the cure . . ."

A leading pharmaceutical company in 1987 had generously offered to donate a very effective medicine (tablets) to the world to eliminate river blindness. The idea is this: when a black fly *vector* (an insect that carries germs) bites an individual infected with the parasite, the fly can then transmit the parasite to the next individual it bites. Only humans carry the infection; if humans aren't infected, the disease will perish. So the plan was to provide these tablets to treat everyone (known as mass drug administration) in the community older than age five years every six months to eliminate the parasite from their bodies and thus stop the spread. The treatments would have to be sustained for many years.

So in 1988 there were many questions about whether these poor and largely indigenous communities in Guatemala would accept the medicine. Working in developing countries, I've become accustomed to cultural differences that often impede the delivery of what the best-intentioned of us believe to be good practice. Issues of communication, trust, and education can be paramount. We needed to understand the people of these communities more fully to determine how to communicate and gain the trust and cooperation needed to get enough people to agree to take the treatment every six months for years and years. Paramount to success was good and sustained treatment coverage of the entire local population.

To understand how to do this, we were visiting terribly impoverished coffee plantations on the slopes of Guatemalan volcanoes, where the rivers cascading down the slopes created perfect breeding grounds for the black flies and river blindness parasites. It was in these areas that blindness was epidemic and more than 80 percent of villagers were infected. With skilled interviewers, we conducted a "knowledge, attitudes, and practices" survey, hoping to find out what health issues were highest on the villagers' list of concerns. Of course, a finding that river blindness was a significant concern to the villagers would predict a greater chance of success with our mass treatment approach; if river blindness was not a priority for the villagers, we would have an educational challenge ahead of us. The most important question on the survey: "What do you think are the major health problems in your village?"

Most of the villagers were indigenous peoples; the men spoke Spanish, albeit haltingly, but most of the women spoke only their native Mayan languages. It was a tremendous logistical hurdle to capture the information we sought. We had to design our survey questions well to be sure we posed the kinds of questions that would give us the answers we needed to design the best health educational approach to accompany the mass treatment program.

As the sun was setting one evening, casting an angular orange glow on the small plantation where we were conducting the survey, I sat with the interviewer working with me in a hut with a thatched roof, interviewing a family. I was trying to be inconspicuous, sitting in a corner on an old chair, letting the interviewer do all the work. A mangy dog lay by my side. Kids were running around with almost no clothing, malnourished, with obvious deep skin sores from scabies (another parasitic disease), dodging the chickens that roamed freely around the room nipping at insects on the dirt floor of the hut. This was my seventh or eighth interview on this project, and I was growing accustomed to hearing, in response to our "major health problems" question, diarrhea, worms, pneumonia, and other typical scourges of the developing world. Only a couple of the prior interviewees included river blindness on their priority lists, which made us realize education about the disease would be critical for gaining acceptance of our treatment program.

Sitting in another corner of this tiny hut was an old man. He was tanned, had a white stubble beard, and was dressed in rags like the others. Yet he had subtle nobility about him; he seemed to observe the event distantly. He hadn't said a word as my interviewer questioned others in the family, but I noticed him staring at me from time to time throughout our visit. Whenever I looked back at him, we briefly met eyes. Glaring is not the right word, since I did not think he was hostile toward me, more curious. Finally, after the others had spoken, I returned his gaze and asked in a soft respectful voice, in Spanish, "Señor, what do you believe is the major health problem here?"

He met my gaze and his reply came after a short pause, "*Fijese esta pobreza que no se escapa.*" Translation: "Fix yourself on this poverty that cannot be escaped." Then his face softened and, nodding, he almost seemed to smile at me, as if to say "Here endeth the lesson. Education complete, my son."

It struck me as a lightning bolt, straight between the eyes. Of course I knew that. Lessons are miraculous when you know them already, when it only takes someone to articulate for you what you know. I was so fixated on this one disease, this one effort, that I was lost. Now I was enlightened, and ashamed and humbled by the obviousness of his statement; how could I be so blind to it? My teacher knew I had asked a shallow, stupid question; it was his concise and profound answer that mattered. Speechless, I averted my gaze, nodded and bowed my head. When the interview was over I shook his hand, met his eyes, thanked him, and left, never to see him again.

His face and his answer still haunt me today, and I can call upon the memory of that experience at will, reliving the full emotions, visions, sensations of that very moment.

We international health experts, well-intentioned and highly motivated, wade deep in our weeds of infectious diseases theory and infection control strategy, studying patterns and trend lines of illnesses and deaths in isolated villages. Yet this wizened man had found a perch above it all from which he could see the big picture and teach us doctors a lesson.

As I have often reflected on this wonderful event, the lines of an Eagles song always come to mind:

"An old man told me
Tryin' to scold me . . ."

I guess he was softly scolding me, as a good teacher might, to get that tension to pass that message to the obtuse student. Of course river blindness was a major health concern in Guatemala and on this coffee plantation—as were diarrhea, pneumonia, typhoid, malaria, and hepatitis. But the major health problem, above all else, was inescapable poverty. Imagine: poverty so great and powerful, so all-encompassing and ever-present, the root cause of all infection and perhaps all illness. A downward spiral generated a spiritual hopelessness; utter despair for a future that can be no more than that hut, and all that it encompassed. Cure my poverty, and you will cure me.

As I write this essay, I am also completing my report for a medical journal on the successful elimination of river blindness from Guatemala. One hundred years after a Guatemalan was the first to discover river blindness, that nation has requested verification of elimination of the disease from the World Health Organization. The juxtaposition of these two writing projects, the eradication report and this essay on "the real major medical problem," is powerful. On the one hand, I'm excited to have reached this stage of our river blindness mission, to have achieved the goal we set out to achieve nearly three decades years ago. On the other hand, when seen from the perch of that old man so many years ago, our accomplishments are only a small piece of the dilemma. That old man, if he is living, doesn't have river blindness to worry about any more. But so what? The job is yet undone; so much more to do. Sweet—yet bitter—success. As a father he warned me of the height of the mountain that I was daring to climb. Keep heart and keep sanity.

"Whoa, son, don't wade too deep in Bitter Creek."

How miraculous his single sentence was for me, and how much it taught me! I am a different person and different physician because of my visit to the old man's hut in 1988.

I encourage my public health students to expose themselves to similar uncomfortable situations, to be attentive and learn from the most humble of those we have the opportunity to meet and interact with in our profession. What we will find will be unexpected insight and wisdom. What they tell us will miraculously reenergize our commitments and renew our strengths. It will plant a seed that will sprout as motivation for the next difficult step in our mission to help leave a better world.

Step back from the statistics and data to find a perch, and try to see the big picture. That old man did just that by scolding me and warning me, all at the same time.

The results of our 1991 survey where I met the old sage can be found at:

F. Richards, R. Klein, C. Gonzales Peralta, R. Zea Flores, G. Zea Flores, and J. Castro Ramírez. Knowledge, attitudes, and perceptions (KAP) of onchocerciasis: A survey among residents in an endemic area in Guatemala targeted for mass chemotherapy with ivermectin. *Social Science and Medicine* 1991; 32: 1275–1281.

The results of our declaration of river blindness elimination in the Central Endemic Zone:

Frank Richards Jr, Nidia Rizzo, Carlos Enrique Diaz Espinoza, Zoraida Morales Monroy, Carol Guillermina Crovella Valdez, Renata Mendizabal de Cabrera, Oscar de Leon, Guillermo Zea-Flores, Mauricio Sauerbrey, Alba Lucia Morales, Dalila Rios, Thomas R. Unnasch, Hassan K. Hassan, Robert Klein, Mark Eberhard, Ed Cupp, and Alfredo Domínguez. One hundred years after its discovery in Guatemala by Rodolfo Robles, *Onchocerca volvulus* transmission has been eliminated from the Central Endemic Zone. *American Journal of Tropical Medicine and Hygiene* 2015 Dec; 93(6): 1295–1304.

For more information on river blindness and our efforts to eradicate this disease: *http://www.cartercenter.org/health/river_blindness/index.html*

The Miracle in
the Middle

Mark F. Cotton, M Med (Paed), PhD

F or a child born almost anywhere in Africa in 2001, and for that matter in many parts of Africa still today, the phrase "medical miracle" is an oxymoron. The cumulative devastations of famine, disease, and dire poverty conspire to make good outcomes a rarity. This is all the more so for children born with AIDS, the rate of which was still growing alarmingly in 2001 before it finally peaked in 2002. That's what makes this baby's story so miraculous.

Little "Anna" was born in 2001 to a mother living in one of the poorest "informal settlements" (dense clusters of thrown-together, ramshackle huts and shacks where the destitute live) in South Africa. Early in life she developed chronic lung disease, a common manifestation of congenital (acquired at birth) AIDS. She was dependent for survival on receiving supplemental oxygen through a tube in her nose attached to an oxygen tank. She could not possibly receive such therapy in her home, a shack without plumbing and electricity. She lived in our hospital for more than three months with no sign that her lungs would ever heal enough to be able to return home. Such is the nature of the AIDS lung disease in babies.

In the hospital, she spent almost every minute of her life lying flat on her back, receiving oxygen. Trying to breathe was her main job—there wasn't energy left for rolling over, or smiling, or playing with a rattle. There also wasn't enough energy left to grow, and she was failing to put on weight. We all loved this little baby—the doctors, nurses, and aides. We took her for walks, along with her oxygen, whenever anyone had a free moment. But the hospital was always understaffed, and there were few free moments. So mostly she just lay there, alert, aware of everyone around her, desperate to develop as a baby, but simply too debilitated by her lung disease and her inability to eat.

We now know that using "triple therapy"—three powerful drugs that treat HIV, the virus that causes AIDS—is the most successful approach to treating patients, including young infants. The first clinical trial of triple therapy for children in South Africa began in 1998 and was funded by a pharmaceutical company. Early results looked very promising, and we began trying to raise independent funds to pay for kids' triple therapy once the clinical trial was over and the pharmaceutical money gone. Thanks to private fundraising efforts led by my wife, Reena, and others, especially HOPE Cape Town, we were able to buy triple therapy for little Anna and a number of other babies that year. The pharmaceutical company gave us a limited grant to buy anti-HIV drugs for the ongoing treatment of the 1998 study patients, of which Anna was not one (she was born in 2001, too late to be included in the study). By a combination of private donations and that grant money, we patched together enough stocks of medicines to treat Anna and the others. But for how long could we continue to afford to treat these babies? We knew that once the money ran out and their therapy ended, their HIV infection would flare, their AIDS would relapse, and they would die.

The results in Anna were nothing short of amazing. True to the impressions we were getting from the 1998 study and from similar research elsewhere about the benefits of triple therapy, Anna dramatically improved. Her lung disease was cured by the anti-HIV drugs—*cured!* She no longer needed oxygen, she gained weight, and she caught up on her developmental milestones. Assessments of the living situation of her biological mother, who was never able to visit her child in the hospital, were bleak. Anna's biological father had deserted the family when he heard his wife and daughter had AIDS. Anna's biological mother found a new partner, but didn't disclose her HIV infection to him, and was now pregnant again. It was clear that a foster home would be needed to provide adequate medical care for Anna, and we found an excellent placement for her. We didn't know how, or for how long, we could afford to pay for her triple therapy, which was lifesaving.

We managed to beg, borrow, and stretch our funding for Anna's and the others' treatments from 2001 to 2004. Then, just as we were confronting the reality that the grant funding was ending and we had run out of private donations, a miracle arrived from the unlikeliest of sources: the government of South Africa announced it would provide free access to triple therapy for all AIDS patients in public clinics. Because of our experience with anti-AIDS drugs for children, our clinic was one of the first to obtain these life-saving medicines for children, with just days to spare before Anna's therapy would have ended.

Anna continued to thrive in every way, receiving her triple therapy in her foster home without interruption, never knowing how close we came to failing her. Sandwiched exactly in the middle between the first clinical trial for children in 1998 (three years before Anna was born), and 2004, the year effective therapy finally became available to all babies born with AIDS in South Africa (but three years after she needed to begin treatment), it wouldn't have seemed as if Anna had much of a chance of survival. Without the anti-HIV medicines, she would have wasted away in the hospital and died of her lung disease.

Instead, thanks to the highly improbable confluence of Good Samaritans' generosity, a grant from a pharmaceutical company, and the government's timely policy change, Anna is a survivor of AIDS in Africa.

Miraculous.

For more about HOPE Cape Town: *http://www.hopecapetown.com*

When the Student Is Ready,
the Teacher Appears

David Addiss, MD, MPH

O n a granite wall in the lobby of the World Health Organization (WHO) headquarters in Geneva, an aspirational vision is inscribed in several languages: "The attainment by *all* peoples of the highest possible level of health." Within this building, and in medical centers, public health agencies, and clinics around the world, an estimated 59 million people in the global health workforce labor to improve the health of *all* people—including some of the most marginalized and neglected populations on earth. The people who benefit from their dedicated efforts may never know—or even be aware of—the millions of global health workers who serve on their behalf. Yet, over the course of time, the results of those efforts are nothing short of miraculous.

At its best, global health represents a massive effort to alleviate and prevent human suffering, without regard to race, religion, nationality, or creed. Those who work in global health aim to improve the health of entire populations. They deal with numbers, graphs, and statistics. They may work in sprawling government agencies or in small volunteer organizations. What motivates this outpouring of compassionate action? What is it that makes this work so deeply meaningful? What is it that sustains the spirits of these workers in the face of overwhelming challenges of disease, poverty, bureaucratic frustrations, political inaction and, at times, insecurity and conflict?

Often it is a personal encounter with a particular individual that has provided the most powerful inspiration. The stories of these encounters, which may have lasted only moments, can sustain an entire career. The content of these stories varies. Community health workers may remember a neighbor or community member who endured a devastating illness with dignity and courage, or they may have borne witness to the life-saving power of a simple intervention, such as oral rehydration. Physicians may recall particular patients whose lives touched theirs, perhaps with a sense of gratitude in having accompanied and been of service to someone who overcame a serious illness. Some of the most poignant stories are "wake-up calls," in which assumptions were challenged and the limitations of the health worker's knowledge or efforts were starkly revealed. My colleague, Frank Richards, beautifully describes such an encounter in another essay in this book ("The Miracle of a Single Sentence"). My story was also a "wake-up call."

During the early 1990s, I was part of a scientific team at the Centers for Disease Control and Prevention (CDC) studying new drug treatments for *lymphatic filariasis* (LF), a disfiguring tropical disease caused by parasitic worms that are spread by mosquitoes. In humans, the adult worms live in the lymphatic vessels, channels that drain excess fluid and waste from body tissues. The damage to these vessels caused by the worms results in swelling of the leg, known as *lymphedema*, in an estimated 14 million people worldwide. As lymphedema progresses to its advanced form, *elephantiasis*, the skin becomes rough, thick, and hard—elephant-like. These changes in the tissue reduce the movement of the affected limbs and the ability of its victims to work. Episodes of pain, inflammation, and high fever, called acute attacks, occur, further damaging the skin and underlying tissue.

The prevailing hypothesis at the time I began in this work was that those horribly painful and debilitating acute attacks were triggered by the body's own reaction to the adult worm, that the progression of lymphedema was due to that abnormal immune response, and that nothing could be done to alter the course of the disease. In many communities where LF is prevalent, lymphedema is considered a mark of shame, a sign of having been cursed; those who develop lymphedema are to be avoided for fear of contagion. People with

LF sometimes consider the social, psychological, and emotional suffering of stigmatization to be worse than the physical suffering it causes.

As I joined the CDC team and began traveling with them to Ste. Croix Hospital in Leogane, Haiti, I was struck by how little we understood about this ancient disease. We began to investigate some of the most perplexing questions about LF by correlating clinical and laboratory findings on individual patients. My role, as the clinician on the team, was to examine patients after my colleagues, laboratory scientists, had tested their blood for the LF parasite. To those who were infected, I gave a standard dose of the recommended medicine, *diethylcarbamazine* (DEC). A very brief encounter with one of these patients changed the course of my life.

It was a hot, humid August night in the outpatient clinic of Ste. Croix Hospital. Toward the end of the evening, a thin young woman, seventeen years old, approached the airless, stifling examination room where I was working. I greeted her and invited her in, noticing that one of her legs was already swollen and the skin was starting to thicken. I learned through a translator that the swelling had begun two to three years earlier and it was getting progressively worse. I was tired. It had been a long day. In a rather perfunctory way, I took measurements of her leg, did a cursory examination of her heart, lungs, and limbs, and checked the laboratory sheet, which told me that, indeed, she was infected with the LF parasite. According to protocol, I measured out the proper number of DEC tablets for her weight, placed them in her open hand, provided a cup of water, and asked her to swallow the pills. I will never forget what happened next.

Instead of closing her hand around the tablets to swallow them, she looked me straight in the eye with a weary look of exasperation and disgust. Holding her gaze, she raised her hand upward, and with a flourish threw the DEC tablets forcefully, angrily, across the floor of the small room. She turned on her heels and marched out of the room. I never saw her again.

I was stunnned and, for a moment, indignant. Didn't she know we were offering her the standard treatment, recommended by the experts at the

WHO, for LF infection? Did she not recognize the efforts our CDC team had made to travel to Haiti and provide what limited care we could? How dare she waste those tablets when other infected patients could have benefited from them! Didn't she know her lymphedema could get worse if her infection was not successfully treated? But the fire in her eyes soon made me realize that she understood, at a level that I had not yet accepted, that our drug treatment, the international "standard of care" from the experts who advised WHO, would do nothing to prevent her acute attacks or her leg from swelling further—nor would it reduce the stigma and social isolation that she was already experiencing. She had been offered pills before, with no effect. She knew that for her, and we would later learn for tens of thousands of other patients as well, DEC alone would not meaningfully change her disease. She was unimpressed by these foreigners who had encouraged her to come to the hospital clinic with the promise of hope, but instead only took her blood for tests, made a few measurements, and offered some pills that would be of little or no benefit. We were wasting her time. She knew she needed more than DEC—we just didn't realize it yet.

An Eastern proverb says that when the student is ready, the teacher appears. This young woman had become my teacher. I could not shake her fierce gaze. She had opened my eyes and forced me to see that our scientific theories, academic publications, and travel to exotic places to do research offered little real hope to her or millions like her. My fundamental assumptions—not just about how LF does what it does, but also about what exactly I thought I was doing—needed serious rethinking.

When the student is ready, the teacher appears. The young Haitian woman prepared me to receive with an open mind the instruction of another teacher. Gerusa Dreyer is a dynamic Brazilian physician whose astute powers of clinical observation and compassionate care for thousands of patients led her to a new understanding of LF. She came to question the dominant theory that acute attacks were caused by the body's own response to the adult worm. To Dr. Dreyer, many of these attacks looked just like common bacterial infections of the tissue known as *cellulitis*. Her research showed that breaks in the skin and sores on the feet and legs allowed bacteria to enter, and that poor drainage through the diseased lymphatic channels allowed the bacteria to flourish. In other words, the disease caused by the worm predisposed the patient to the bacteria, which in turn caused the acute attacks. That's why DEC alone could never work in that young Haitian woman. In her own dramatic way, that's what she was trying to teach me.

If acute attacks were due to bacteria, they might be preventable! Extending her research, Dr. Dreyer showed that progression of lymphedema to elephantiasis could be halted, and in many cases reversed, by a simple regimen of hygiene and skin care (to treat and prevent the breaks in the skin that could allow bacteria to enter), movement, and leg elevation. She organized "Hope Clubs" to teach her patients self-care and to overcome their social and emotional isolation.

I arranged to travel to Recife, Brazil, to visit Dr. Dreyer and to see for myself what she was doing. All too aware that her message of hope went against the grain of what medical scientists thought possible at the time, she insisted on two things before she allowed me to visit. First, I must learn enough Portuguese to converse with and understand the patients as they described their experience. Second, if I was convinced by what I saw, I must promise to do what I could to bring these teachings and practices to Haiti.

A "Hope Club" happened to be scheduled on the day I arrived in Recife. I was astonished by the festive atmosphere and by the palpable sense of empowerment, community, and, yes, hope that pervaded the room. Many of these patients had advanced lymphedema, but they were animated, joyful, engaged. I spent several days in the clinic, learning from Dr. Dreyer's team, speaking with patients, and learning her simple but profound lymphedema self-care techniques.

I was so deeply moved by this experience that I dedicated the next twelve years of my life to this cause. With Dr. Dreyer's help, my colleagues in Haiti established a lymphedema management program there, along with Hope

Clubs and support groups. Together with others, we did studies to demonstrate the effectiveness of these techniques, participated in lymphedema training for health workers around the world, and pushed for this type of care to be considered an integral part of the WHO program to eliminate LF as a public health problem. No longer would we be handing out DEC tablets alone to treat lymphedema or elephantiasis.

It is possible—indeed likely—that I would have done none of this had I not experienced the defiant gaze of the young woman in Haiti. The power of these individual encounters, and the meaning they convey, are a rich source of inspiration for global health action. Global health is a complex, somewhat chaotic system of international agencies, governments, non-governmental organizations, and foundations, often with competing priorities. So much less would be achieved through these organizations were it not for the networks of trust, respect, and—why not say it?—love that join people together in common purpose. The qualities that motivate global action to relieve suffering are so often inspired and nurtured by the memory of a particular encounter with an individual.

During the past several years, what we used to call "international health" has been replaced by "global health," which is grounded in the realization of human interconnectedness. The epidemics of HIV/AIDS, SARS (severe acute respiratory syndrome), and Ebola virus—to name only a few—have shown us how deeply interdependent our health and health systems are. In a real sense, the distinction between global and local has virtually disappeared. For example, Chagas' disease, a parasitic disease spread by bugs that live in thatch roofs and walls, was once limited to Latin America. The debilitating heart failure and premature mortality caused by Chagas' attracted little attention elsewhere. However, with immigration and global travel, Chagas' disease is increasingly recognized as a public health problem in the United States and Europe. What was once a local problem now requires a global solution.

The miracle of global health lies in the power of an individual face, an individual encounter, to transform a heart, change a life, and inspire a career that alleviates human suffering on a global scale. Global health is an expression of this rich interplay between the faces and the numbers, individuals and populations, global and local, the whole and its parts. In the busy day-to-day work of global health, immersed in programs, numbers, and bureaucratic challenges, it is easy to lose sight of the faces. In the words of Catholic theologian Gustavo Gutiérrez, we must continually drink from our own wells. The living memories of our individual stories make possible the refreshing waters of renewal and regeneration.

Spiritual teachers through the ages have pointed toward our human interconnectedness and the need to have compassion for all. To paraphrase the words of Mother Teresa, they teach us to draw the circle of our family ever more widely. Thousands of years ago, when humans still lived in small bands of hunter-gatherers, such a universal vision would have seemed incomprehensible, unnecessary, and even dangerous. It is still not an easy vision to practice. However, we now realize that adopting this vision is essential for the future of the planet. Global health is in the vanguard of carrying forward, in practical ways, this universal spiritual vision. It is this vision that is inscribed on the wall at WHO and inspires the 59 million people dedicated to global health care.

The face of the young Haitian woman with lymphedema remains with me still. I do not know what became of her. Did she ever benefit from the lymphedema management programs that were established in Haiti? I don't know. I do know that, if she has children, they are growing up free from the threat of LF, as are millions more around the world, thanks to the efforts of a vast army of community health workers, government health officials, and non-governmental organizations. And now, hundreds of thousands of people with lymphedema in dozens of LF-endemic countries are learning the self-care techniques that Dr. Dreyer developed and taught.

I am grateful for what the young Haitian woman taught me and grateful for the millions of people from all walks of life whose courage, wisdom, and insight continue to inspire the field of global health.

To learn more about the work of global health, see:

Koplan, J. P., Bond, T. C., Merson, M. H., Reddy, K. S., Rodriguez, M. H., Sewankambo, N. K., & Wasserheit, J. N. (2009). Towards a common definition of global health. *Lancet*, 373, 1993–1995.

Addiss, D.G. (2013b) Global elimination of lymphatic filariasis: A mass uprising of compassion. *PLoS Negl Trop Dis.* 7(8): e2264. doi:10.1371/journal.pntd.0002264.

Addiss, D.G. Globalization of compassion: The example of global health. In: Gill S and Cadman D, eds. *Why love matters: Values in governance.* New York, NY: Peter Lang Publishing 2016; 107–119

8

Miracles in Their Own Time

As medicine advances, yesterday's miracles can become today's expected outcomes. Often, a miraculous event in its time accelerates our progress toward turning the miraculous into the mundane. The results of new research, the advent of new technology, and the accumulation of clinical experience all contribute to that transition.

The stories in this chapter reflect on miracles in the context of their period in history and with an eye toward the future of medicine. Indeed, when in the course of history a medical event occurs often determines the outcome of that event. The first essay is the dramatic firsthand description of Patrick Kennedy, the premature baby born to President John F. and Jackie Kennedy. Even the most powerful man in the world could not call forth a miracle before its time.

Other essays reflect on the evolution of medicine over time and illustrate the striking transition from miracle to everyday occurrence. Examples include heart disease, sudden infant death syndrome, inborn errors of metabolism, AIDS, breast cancer, and battlefield medicine.

It is most rewarding to know that as we push the envelope with each new advance in medicine, ample room for new miracles emerges.

DATE OF EVENT: AUGUST 7–9, 1963

President Kennedy's Baby: Born Too Soon for the Miracle

Richard Johnston Jr. MD

I t was the summer of 1963, and I had begun the third year of my pediatrics residency training in July at Boston Children's Hospital, Harvard Medical School. John F. Kennedy had been elected President of the United States in November 1960 and had assumed office in January 1961. He and his wife, Jacqueline Lee Bouvier Kennedy (Jackie), were parents of a daughter, Caroline, five years old that summer, and a son, John Jr. ("John John"), who was two.

My July assignment was in the newborn nursery at the obstetrical hospital, Boston Lying-In. It was a busy nursery, housing babies born to mothers at that hospital. Most of the babies were normal and healthy, but some had birth defects or were born prematurely, before a completed pregnancy. Babies needing surgery or special care were transferred to a nursery at Children's Hospital across the street.

One of the most common and most feared complications of prematurity was a lung disorder called *hyaline membrane disease* (HMD), now known as *respiratory distress syndrome*. The condition is characterized by a glassy coating (membrane) in the baby's air sacs that obstructs the normal transfer of oxygen from the lungs to the circulating blood. Affected babies develop rapid, shallow, and noisy breathing, and a frightening blue-gray skin color as they struggle to take in enough air. Without treatment the affected baby is caught in a desperate battle that can end in death if his respiratory muscles and energy reserves wear down before the lungs improve.

There was no effective treatment for this disorder that summer, nor was there clear understanding of its cause. We knew HMD was more common in babies born by cesarean section and in boys. No racial or ethnic group was spared. My wife had delivered our first son nine months earlier, thankfully at full term. I knew well the intense feelings of expectation and anxiety evoked by the birth process, and caring as a resident for a preterm baby with HMD was a sad, frustrating, and anxious experience for me.

Early in my assignment at Boston Lying-In, I learned that the pediatricians there had experimented with placing several HMD babies that they felt would otherwise die into a high-pressure (hyperbaric) chamber located beneath the garden that was part of the Children's Hospital grounds. Under increased pressure, the oxygen given a baby could pass easily through the obstructed lungs into the circulation. The chamber was normally used at Children's to keep blood oxygen levels high during complicated heart surgery and as treatment for certain types of severe infection. The babies with HMD treated experimentally in this chamber quickly lost their blue color and relaxed their struggle as their blood oxygen reached levels several-fold higher than those of a normal infant. In a matter of hours, however, the babies' condition had rapidly worsened, their breathing had again become shallow, and all had died.

On the first of August, I moved across the street to the oncology service at Children's Hospital. By August 7, I was embedded in my responsibilities on this new service when we heard that Jackie Kennedy had delivered a boy by caesarean section at an Air Force hospital near the Kennedy family compound on Cape Cod. He was Patrick Bouvier Kennedy, born five and a half weeks prematurely, weighing four pounds, ten and a half ounces, with HMD; and, he was on his way by ambulance to Children's Hospital. Shortly after his arrival at Children's, the President landed by helicopter in the Fenway, a park area near the hospital. It was clear on Patrick's arrival that he was in severe respiratory distress.

Early the next morning I was standing in the doorway of the nursery when the President came around a corner and nodded a quiet greeting. There was no smile. I think I had enough presence to respond, but I remember clearly the sense that I had been momentarily stunned. I thought it remarkable at the time that he was alone. He had been accompanied by very few Secret Service agents when he entered the hospital the evening before. Times were different then, but the lax security around the President and his apparent lack of concern for his safety would cost him his life three and a half months later.

Patrick's condition deteriorated over the course of that day, and it appeared that he would die unless something more effective could be done. Hyperbaric oxygen delivery was deemed the only remaining hope, and he was placed in the chamber late that day. As with the other babies, his color returned to normal quickly, his respiratory distress dissipated, and his condition stabilized—until early the next day when his struggle returned and he died. A fellow resident told me that the President's brother Bobby, the United States Attorney General at the time, had sat at the entrance to the hyperbaric oxygen chamber and grilled the residents as they came in and out caring for the baby.

I remember that Children's Hospital was quiet and sad that morning. It felt to me that we had failed a fine young mother and father. There was no miracle here, not even for a President's son.

Research that had begun a few years before Patrick's birth had indicated that HMD was the result of deficiency of a substance in premature babies' lungs. Subsequent basic research identified that substance as *surfactant*, a slippery lipid-protein mix that allows the lung's air sacs to open and fill with air. Surfactant develops in the later stages of pregnancy; the smaller the premature baby, the greater the surfactant deficiency. Clinical research that followed the basic science defined the most effective preparations and strategies to replace the missing surfactant.

I believe that "medical miracles" have a biologic basis that can be discovered through research. Discovering the basic causes of disease leads to their treatment. Even babies born much more prematurely than Patrick Kennedy are alive today because of the research that came too late to save a President's son.

Patrick was born too soon, five and a half weeks before full term maturity would have made the risk of HMD negligible, and a few decades before the product of basic science and clinical research would have easily saved his life.

DATE OF EVENT: DECEMBER 1944, AND 2013

Battlefield Miracles, from Generation to Generation

Paul A. Skudder, MD

Decem ber 16, 1944, began the Battle of the Bulge in bitter, near-arctic conditions of an unusually harsh Northern European winter. The German *Wehrmacht* (war machine) waited for near-impenetrable fog, snow, and freezing rain to send almost a quarter million soldiers, backed by all the panzer tanks the Russians hadn't obliterated on the Eastern front, into a poorly defended segment of the American lines in Belgium, just west of Germany.

General George Patton and the United States Third Army's heroism in saving the thousands of men cut off in the city of Bastogne, and the massacre of American POWs in Malmedy, are well known. Reversal of this attack took over a month, at a cost of 19,000 American soldiers' lives, over a third of the death toll of ten-plus years of fighting in Vietnam, and many times the number killed in Afghanistan and Iraq in the recent wars. Seventy-thousand other American GIs survived being wounded in those bitter winter conditions. A portion of them were treated for ghastly wounds at the 16th General Hospital, a freezing cold tent facility of 1,000-plus beds located just north of the "Bulge" itself, outside Liege, Belgium, near the German border.

Among the GIs in the 16th General Hospital was a twenty-year-old high school dropout serving as a private in the Medical Corps, doing the grunt work needed to keep a "M*A*S*H" military field hospital running. So moved was this young man that he regarded the surgeons working to save the thousands of wounded with religious awe, and what they achieved as miracles.

Following the war a changed young man finished high school, and the GI Bill allowed a college and medical school education to follow, leading to a civilian career on the surgical faculty of a major university medical center.

That young man was my dad. Could he have foreseen the future, and what his experience in that miserable winter would lead to?

✧ ✧ ✧

Sixty-nine years later, a twenty-one-year-old soldier, far from his home in Tennessee, stepped on an *IED* (improvised explosive device) in Helmand Province of Afghanistan. America was back at war, and once again U.S. soldiers were taking casualties. Germany was again at the heart of the treatment of battlefield wounded.

The soldier collapsed, blood streaming from his legs, exposed bones and muscle dangling. He is one of hundreds, even thousands. These so-called improvised devices are actually very sophisticated. They have radio controlled triggers, pressure triggers like a land mine, or wire-controlled triggers; these are major explosive devices that have destroyed many vehicles.

A field paramedic embedded in the soldier's unit provides first aid. The soldier is promptly evacuated to the nearest Forward Operating Base, where emergency surgery is done. Dead tissue is removed, which unfortunately includes most of his left leg. There's dead tissue in the right leg as well, but notwithstanding multiple broken bones, it appears that limb is salvageable. Hemorrhage is stopped. Bolts are drilled through broken bones, and an external "erector set" is used to manipulate the bones into position to allow healing to begin. Infection is addressed with antibiotics, and most importantly through aggressive surgical removal of dead tissue.

The patient is transfused with blood, and soon thereafter is flown by helicopter to a combat surgical hospital. Again, he undergoes surgery. More unhealthy tissue is removed. Sterile fluids and antibiotics are used to flush out foreign material from the wounds: grit and grime, fragments of clothing, fragments of weapons. Sophisticated suction dressings are applied. Fluids and antibiotics are administered. The patient is carefully evaluated for associated injuries to his brain, eardrums, lungs, heart, kidneys, and other vital structures.

A giant C-17 Globemaster Air Force transport plane lowers a huge trapdoor under its tail. An ambulance bus nearly drives up this ramp, but it stops and its rear doors are opened. Injured soldiers from the Combat Surgical Hospital are carried aboard by hand stretchers. The belly of this plane is not filled with rows of seats, although there are seats around the walls, facing the center of the airliner. In the center are layered racks for stretchers, accompanied by equipment to allow artificial breathing, transfusions, intravenous fluid administration, cardiac support, and other services consistent with an intensive care unit (ICU). From the back of the ambulance bus our injured soldier is one of those carried aboard the Globemaster by uniformed personnel. His lower body is covered in bandages and adorned by the metallic orthopedic devices that have been drilled through the bones of his remaining leg to repair the shattered bones. His stretcher is fastened into one of the racks, and the plane lifts off, accompanied by nurses and physicians specially trained for the challenges of intensive patient care at 30,000 feet.

Seven hours and thousands of miles later, at Ramstein Air Base in Germany, the scene is repeated in reverse. The stretchers come off the Globemaster, and are loaded into the ambulance buses that are backed up to the rear ramp of the plane. The "walking wounded" follow down the ramp, and all are transported to Landstuhl Regional Medical Center. This is America's largest overseas hospital and serves military and State Department personnel stationed throughout Europe, Asia, and Africa. Since the beginning of Operation Enduring Freedom in Afghanistan, and throughout related operations in Iraq, Landstuhl has been the primary site of treatment of major injuries arising in these war zones. American soldiers and their comrades from coalition countries have been arriving there daily.

The hospital is staffed by full-time military physicians on active duty, reservists called up to active duty, as well as by civilian volunteer physicians giving their time and skills to allow the Army to send additional uniformed active-duty physicians "down-range" into the war zone.

As I—the son of that Army private who saw the miracles, and tragedies, of combat medicine in the cold winter of 1944—stand among my fellow surgeons awaiting the injured soldier from Tennessee, I reflect on how powerfully and proudly my father's experience has been passed to another generation.

We at Landstuhl know what to expect. It is surely not the first time. The flight plan from Bagram Airbase in Afghanistan has been transmitted to the ICU at Landstuhl; arrival time is precisely known. The patient's records fly through the electronic ether and the details of physician reports and care provided at each step of the way flash on to the computer screen of the ICU in Germany hours before the patient's arrival. The next steps in his care are planned. Appropriate personnel are ready and waiting as the young man is lifted off the ambulance bus at the Landstuhl emergency entrance.

The young soldier is wheeled into the ICU. We examine him and compare our findings with the information transmitted from down-range. Large wounds, both legs, and one leg missing. Genital wounds, the blast from below. They're open, bones exposed, but the wounds have been well cared for en route to us. There is no active bleeding, yet inevitably some debris still accumulated in the depths of the wounds.

Back to the operating room. The remaining debris, Afghani soil, and metallic fragments are removed. All living tissue is left in place. Detailed protocols have been developed by the Army Institute for Surgical Research for care of these injuries, based on careful analysis of thousands of such victims. The pattern of wounds in each soldier is electronically recorded, as is the treatment and outcome to find the most effective paradigm to treat each constellation of injuries. Newly enlisted active-duty physicians, reservists called up, and we volunteer surgeons all have access to the same best practice protocols; nobody needs to reinvent the wheel.

We administer antibiotics and vaccines for infections we don't see in the West; this, too, has been driven by detailed analysis of years of experience with such complex medical and surgical cases. Pain medication, psychological support, physical therapy, and attentive nursing care all working together for each soldier as an individual.

Our Tennessee soldier gets stronger each day, less pain medicine, cleaner wounds. Plans for reconstruction and rehabilitation are being made, and thoughts turn to home. Thousands of miles farther must be traveled. It's back to the C-17 Globemaster, with its four large jet engines on a wing over the fuselage, lifting the giant belly of the plane—a belly full of stretchers surrounded by specialists, and the "walking wounded" in the seats with their backs to the outside walls. Another seven or eight hours, this time to Andrews Air Force Base and Walter Reed Medical Center. Then they will be closer to home where a family from Tennessee can visit, and further efforts can be made in reconstructing wounds, supporting families, and rebuilding lives.

By the time soldiers reach Germany, most know they're going to survive. Miraculously, and a true tribute to the infrastructure of military medicine, 98 percent of those who make it off the battlefield to the nearest Forward Operating Base alive will survive. If the soldier is not killed on the battlefield, his or her chances of survival are now overwhelmingly good.

The young private in Germany decades earlier who witnessed surgeons working battlefield miracles would have loved to see this new day. During his time, in World War II, only about 20 percent of those who were injured on the battlefield survived, and that was a great improvement from the first World War thanks to the introduction of antibiotics.

Ours is a world in seemingly perpetual conflict. Thankfully, since my dad's days in that World War II military field hospital, the odds for soldiers have improved with each conflict. By the Korean War, surgeons were mastering the repair of major blood vessel injuries (which became the basis for heart bypass surgery throughout the world soon afterward). Many advances grew out of the Vietnam experience, among which was the recognition of *Da Nang lung*, a lethal fluid buildup in the lungs that follows injury or infection. Since that time, the treatment of this problem, now known as *adult respiratory distress syndrome* (ARDS), has become a key part of ICU care of patients throughout the world. ARDS affects hundreds of thousands of patients every year who have never been on a battlefield or in a war—yet it was on the battlefield where we learned to recognize and treat that condition. The current level of care our soldiers—and, for that matter, our civilians—receive is built on the shoulders of past soldiers and their battlefield caregivers.

Before flying home to his family, the young soldier from Tennessee expresses profound gratitude to those of us caring for him. I share with him the stories of battlefield miracles performed by generations of physicians and nurses before me—miracles that paved the way for what we can accomplish today. For me, these stories began years before I was born, with the experiences of a young soldier from an earlier generation, a private on the German front in the bitter winter of '44.

DATE OF EVENT: 1973

Safe to Sleep

Henry Sondheimer, MD

I t was a dark and rainy night.... Well, it really *was* a dark and rainy night, and in Northern Arizona where it only rains seven or eight inches a year, that was pretty unusual. I was working at a small, thirty-eight bed hospital on the Hopi Reservation about 250 miles from Phoenix and 80 miles from Winslow, Arizona, where we bought our groceries. We had seven doctors, all Anglo, and about forty nurses, almost all Hopi and Navajo. Our group of doctors had been there for seven months by the time this January night came around so the nurses were familiar with all of us and, probably more importantly, we had the sense that they liked and respected our group of outsiders on their homeland—or at least we hoped they did.

Probably the best strategic decision our group of doctors made was that we would have the on-call doctor sleep in the hospital. This had been a major bone of contention among the group that preceded us. In the end, they had slept at their houses in the government compound two miles away and the nurses didn't like that. The hospital wasn't extremely busy at night, but there was a delivery almost every night and the small ER on the ground floor always had some action: a sick child, a car accident, or just an adult wanting to refill medications. The seven of us were all very young, no one being more than two years out of medical school. Most of the group had done a year of family medicine training, one guy had done two years of internal medicine, and my wife and I had each done two years of pediatrics. No one had formal training in obstetrics and gynecology, surgery, or orthopedics, although we had 250 deliveries each year, fractures, and other orthopedic events regularly. The occasional need for a surgeon always meant an ambulance ride for the patient to the bigger Indian Health Service hospitals seventy miles east and west of us. Over time, we each picked up the skills of at least one of the required specialties that we knew our patients needed but for which we had no formal training: diabetes clinic, TB clinic, field outreach health delivery, etc. I became a regular at prenatal and postpartum clinics.

So that brings us to January. I was on call, had gone home to the compound for dinner, returned in time to see two adults in the ER and deliver a baby, and was finally tucked away into our call room on the second floor of the hospital. I know I was asleep because, when the pediatric nurse called me, I was a little disoriented and didn't at first understand what she was concerned about: "The baby doesn't look good."

What did that mean, "... doesn't look good"? Back in residency at the university hospital last summer I would have expected a lot more detail from the nurse. The baby's temperature, heart rate, and blood pressure. Has he urinated, had bowel movements? But in Hopiland less talk was more. I knew she wouldn't have woken me if she hadn't been concerned, so I held my tongue from all those questions I might have asked six months earlier and jumped out of bed.

And she was right, the baby didn't look good. He was three months old, Navajo, cute as a button. One of my partners had admitted him early the previous morning for pneumonia. Coughing, a few crackles in the chest, and an X-ray that was suggestive of pneumonia, but not overly concerning. He had appropriately sent the baby upstairs to the pediatrics unit. It was probably a viral pneumonia, my partner had written, and he was probably right. It was winter and respiratory viruses were rampant on the reservation. So why didn't the baby look good? I wasn't sure. His temperature was just 100 degrees Fahrenheit, not very high at all. But his color was pale. His blood pressure was good and his heart rate was 104, a little slow but he was sleeping, so probably okay. I listened to his lungs. I kept listening to his lungs. I couldn't hear any signs of pneumonia—and then it struck me. I couldn't hear anything at all—*because he wasn't breathing*. He wasn't breathing!

I turned to the nurse, "Is he breathing?" At first she thought so. I was awake now, adrenaline-fueled. I looked at my watch, at the second hand. I decided I wasn't going to panic. So I watched him, watched him for one full minute. Sixty seconds is a long time when you don't know what's going on. He breathed only twice. Normal babies breathe twenty-four to thirty times a minute, babies with pneumonia are supposed to breathe even faster. I stimulated him, pushed a little on his breast bone, he breathed three or four times in response, but then he slowed back down again. We didn't have the standard heart rate and breathing monitors every hospital off the reservation had. I asked the nurse to recheck his pulse. Still good. It was just his breathing, or lack thereof, that was failing.

I then realized I was looking at a case of impending *sudden infant death syndrome*, or SIDS, or "crib death." Babies who die silently in their sleep, in their cribs. Tragically, these cases are almost always discovered too late, after a baby has already completely stopped breathing for too long to resuscitate. A parent's worst nightmare. This child was on his way to stopping breathing completely, and then to being a crib death. But here he was in front of me, and I certainly wasn't going to let him die. Of course we also didn't have an infant ventilator (breathing machine), so there would be no use putting a tube down his throat to breathe for him the way I learned to during my training. My guess is that even if we had a ventilator we probably wouldn't have had a tube the right size anyway. This wasn't University Hospital.

So there we were, the nurse and I. It was 2:00 AM, very dark and rainy outside, and it's just the two of us and this baby who was trying to become a statistic. And then the nurse turned around, went to the work station, and brought me a nine-inch length of twine. She put it around the baby's ankle, tied a slip knot, and passed it to me. I was catching on by now, so I knotted the metal end of my reflex hammer to the end of the rope. I pulled on the ankle, gently, and the child breathed. I did that every ten seconds or so for about an hour and a half. I wasn't sleepy at all. Every few minutes the nurse would come in and I'd stop stimulating the baby, and we would count his respirations. Slowly they came back up, maybe six or eight per minute at first, but a lusty thirty after ninety minutes. And then he was fine, coughing and acting like he had viral pneumonia, which he did, now with a 101 degrees Fahrenheit temperature. Infections can trigger SIDS. He had passed the crucial moments when his breathing would have stopped entirely. He went on to a full recovery from his pneumonia with no further interruptions of breathing.

I've thought about this night for many years now. It was my miracle that I got to save a child who I am sure would have died of SIDS. And it was the nurse's miracle that she recognized there was something wrong with this baby and stayed by my side through the night. And it was a miracle for the baby and his parents, as well. In recent times, babies like this with "near SIDS," those with slowed breathing or dangerously long gaps between breaths, are sent home from emergency rooms or hospital nurseries with *apnea* monitors. Apnea means lack of breathing, and such monitors can be managed by families of at-risk babies at home. There were no home monitors in 1973. We didn't even have a monitor *in the hospital* for our patient; yet his breathing came back to normal and he was able to go home shortly thereafter without further problems.

But that's not the end of the story. SIDS wasn't even recognized as a distinct medical entity until 1969. In 1974, a year after our little miracle baby, Congress passed the Sudden Infant Death Syndrome Act, recognizing SIDS as a public health threat and directing funds for research. At that time, no one knew the causes or risk factors for SIDS. The first true breakthroughs didn't happen for another decade when *epidemiologists*, scientists who study large populations of people, discovered an association between a baby's sleep position and the risk of SIDS. They discovered that putting a baby to sleep on his back dramatically reduced the risk of SIDS compared with babies who slept on their tummies. A hard sleeping surface was also shown to be protective. In 1994, the Surgeon General of the United States issued a policy statement recommending babies sleep on their backs or sides. This became the "Back to Sleep" public education campaign. (Subsequently, side sleeping has also been shown to be associated with a risk for SIDS, making back sleeping the only recommended position.)

In retrospect, the Navajo parents on our Indian reservation may have been well ahead of their time, and well ahead of other Indian Health Service locations. We had no cases of SIDS occurring in Navajo homes that I can recall or ever heard about (notwithstanding the near-SIDS case I just described). It has since dawned on me that every Navajo baby, probably for hundreds of years, has slept on a board, on his or her back, beginning the day they are born. Back to Sleep. In contrast, other Native American cultures, and other reservations, had very high rates of SIDS. In 2002 and 2003, the National Institutes of Health began educational programs directed specifically at high-risk Native American communities.

The SIDS prevention campaign, now named Safe to Sleep, continues across the world. Dramatic decreases in the rates of SIDS have been achieved in countries where the educational campaign has been introduced, including the United States and including Native American lands within the U.S.

Maybe our miracle baby survived the night and beyond because the nurse and I turned him on his back to pull his ankle with the twine and reflex hammer. Maybe the miracle was that he was seen the day before for viral pneumonia, alerting his mother to a problem and prompting her to venture out on this rainy night when the baby "just didn't look right." Or maybe it was just all of our good fortunes to be there together, in the right place and just in time.

For more about SIDS and safe sleep for babies, see:

National Institutes of Health "Safe to Sleep" website: *https://www.nichd.nih.gov/sts/Pages/default.aspx*

DATE OF EVENT: 1979

The Vitamin That Worked Wonders

Mortimer Poncz, MD

Baby Isadora came to our neonatal intensive care unit with massive diarrhea and in heart failure. She was the second child for these parents, immigrants from a small town in Europe. Their first child had died in infancy of unknown causes; it wasn't long before we discovered the reason for that child's death as well as for Isadora's life-threatening problems.

I was in my fellowship training in hematology at the time, and we were asked to evaluate Isadora for severe *megaloblastic anemia*. Anemia means low red blood cell count, and megaloblastic means that the red blood cells she did have were much too large. The anemia contributed to her heart failure;

having too few red cells, and ineffectively large ones at that, made the heart work much too hard to provide oxygen to the rest of the body. But she also had a poorly functioning heart even after transfusing her with healthy donor red cells.

When I first saw Isadora, she was terribly sick—wasting away from malnutrition due to her diarrhea, and bloated from her heart failure. We hurriedly did testing on her blood and her bone marrow (where the blood is made) and discovered her anemia was due to severe deficiency of a B vitamin called folic acid. Folic acid is essential for nutrition, for making normal cells (including blood cells), and for normal development of the nervous system. Normally, there is enough folic acid in a baby's diet of milk to sustain her, but for some reason Isadora wasn't absorbing the vitamin from her gastrointestinal tract, explaining her severe diarrhea. She was clearly dying in front of our eyes, and it was now apparent her sibling had previously died of the same condition.

At the time, there were a few cases described in the world's medical literature of newborn babies with failure to absorb folic acid. Disappointingly, most of these babies died, and the two or three who had survived were left with severe brain damage, calcifications in the brain, difficult-to-control seizures, and mental retardation. Realizing Isadora's intestines were not absorbing folic acid, we tried giving the vitamin to her with shots. But even if we could get enough vitamin into her by that route, we still had to determine if the folic acid was getting to her brain where it was critical for a normal neurological outcome. It was known that for folic acid to reach the brain it needed to cross the *blood-brain barrier*, a tight layer of cells in the smallest blood vessels of the brain that prevents certain substances from reaching the brain. So we did a spinal tap, a procedure to withdraw a small amount of *cerebrospinal fluid* (CSF), the fluid bathing the brain and spinal cord, to measure the levels of folic acid. We sent the specimen to a research laboratory in the Bronx, New York, which was the only lab in the country at the time testing CSF for folic acid levels. We discovered she had virtually no folic acid in her CSF—a situation which would lead to severe brain damage even if we were able to save her life by treating her anemia and heart failure with the injections.

At this point, I hypothesized that perhaps Isadora and others like her must have had two barriers to folic acid penetration—the one we knew about in her gastrointestinal tract, and another barrier blocking folic acid uptake into the brain. I needed to find a way to get folic acid into her brain (injections into the brain itself would be much too dangerous to give on a daily basis and local concentrated folic acid could itself cause seizures). Reviewing the chemistry of folic acid, I recalled that a related molecule called folinic acid had many of the properties of folic acid but also had a modification of its chemical structure that might allow it to bypass the blood-brain barrier. Folinic acid had been used (and is still used) in cancer therapy, but had never been tried in the very rare type of folic acid deficiency that was killing Isadora.

With her parents' permission, I transferred Isadora to a special research unit at our hospital. There, with the approval of the hospital's human experiment review committee and the consent of her parents, we administered folinic acid to her by shots, carefully monitoring her for side effects. I stayed overnight with her to do three spinal taps following the doses of folinic acid, and arranged with the same laboratory in the Bronx to measure the levels of folic acid in her spinal fluid. If the folinic acid was reaching her brain, the levels of folic acid in her CSF should rise—and they did! I was beyond ecstatic, truly feeling as if I had found a mechanism to not only save this little baby's life, but to also give her the opportunity to grow up intellectually intact and have a full life.

We put Isadora on a regimen of once daily shots of folinic acid. Her diarrhea resolved, as did her anemia and heart failure. Most importantly, as she grew up, we anxiously had her tested and retested to follow her neurologic development and quality of life. We published her case in the medical literature as well as two follow-up reports describing her excellent progress as she went to college and then went on to marry and have two children of her own.

Isadora represented the first cure of this severe form of folic acid deficiency, the first patient to not only survive but with no brain damage. Just as importantly, she hopefully represents the last child who will ever suffer from this rare disorder. Occasionally cases of this type of severe folic acid deficiency still occur. Since our report of this case, it has become standard to treat all such cases as we did for Baby Isadora. And, as with Isadora, the outcomes have been excellent.

Her disease is genetic (inherited), but it requires both parents to be carriers of this very rare defective gene. Isadora's parents were obviously both carriers, but Isadora's husband was not and their children are entirely normal. The defective gene responsible for this disorder has also been identified in part because of our studies of Isadora. It is called the "proton-coupled folate transporter gene."

The care of this baby, who is now, amazingly, a young lady, has contributed greatly to science and to the understanding of how this B vitamin, folic acid, works in the body.

It clearly works wonders.

The original report of this baby's treatment, as published in the medical literature, can be found here:

Poncz M, Colman N, Herbert V, Schwartz E, Cohen AR. Therapy of congenital folate malabsorption. 1981 *J Pediatr.* Jan;98(1):76–9.

The follow-up reports and identification of the responsible gene can be found here:

Poncz M, Cohen. Long-term treatment of congenital folate malabsorption. A. *J Pediatr.* 1996 Dec; 129(6): 948.

Min SH, Oh SY, Karp GI, Poncz M, Zhao R, Goldman ID. The clinical course and genetic defect in the PCFT gene in a 27-year-old woman with hereditary folate malabsorption. *J Pediatr.* 2008 Sep; 153(3): 435–7.

DATE OF EVENT: 1980s–2010s

The Thirty-Year Miracle

Kenneth G. Adams, MD

I am not a big believer in miracles, but please indulge me in some philosophical rambling about the term. Is there really such a thing as a "miracle"? Moses crossing the Red Sea might be explained by his knowledge of weather patterns. The "burning bush" due to a spontaneous brush fire. The "miracle of flight" by the Wright brothers occurred after much studying, observation, and numerous flight trials. I line up more on the side of Thomas Edison, who famously stated that genius is "One percent inspiration and 99 percent perspiration." In the medical field, we all "perspire" a lot. And, sometimes, miracles are the result.

Years ago I consulted on a patient in a local hospital's intensive care unit. He was in a prolonged coma from complications of heart disease. His family was very astute medically and understood the limited chance he had for any recovery whatsoever. For weeks I advised the family to be very pessimistic about recovery. Then he somehow regained consciousness for a few days, talked with me and his family—only to spiral down again.

I have no explanation for how this all happened. Surely his family thought it a miracle that they were able to spend quality time with him before his death, time they never thought they'd have. But the intensive care treatments we were able to provide in terms of blood pressure and breathing support—the "perspiration"—had to have helped, right? Exactly how and why they helped so dramatically for a few days just before his death, and not at all before that or after that, well, I can't really say.

Then there's "broken heart syndrome." We all know stories of someone who passed away a short time after their spouse of many years died. My wife's grandparents died within a week of each other after more than fifty years of marriage. They were reliant upon each other. After all these years of perspiration— expert doctors and scientists trying to figure out what happens in these cases—there was finally some inspiration from specialists in Japan. This syndrome now has a name and an explanation. It's called *takotsubo cardiomyopathy*. It occurs in situations of great stress. One of my patients entered her home, found her husband dead and proceeded to develop takotsubo cardiomyopathy. It has all the markings of a heart attack but is different. There is usually no evidence of blockage in the coronary (heart) arteries the way there is for typical heart attacks. And the hearts in these "broken-hearted" patients are, for lack of a better term, *broken*. More precisely, they have the characteristic shape of a *takotsubo*, the Japanese word meaning octopus pot (a type of trap used to catch octopuses; the octopus crawls into the pot and can't get out, with only a part of the creature protruding from the opening of the pot). There is ballooning (protruding) of the entire left ventricle (the main pumping chamber of the heart), except for the base (the "pot"). On imaging studies, it looks like an octopus pot. Takotsubo cardiomyopathy seems to be stress-induced. No one understands how the heart muscle weakens under stress, but the real miracle here is that most patients recover fully within months. How does the muscle strengthen again? My patient, the one who found her deceased husband, fully recovered her heart strength and function. If only we could harness this miracle of heart muscle recovery and use it in other situations.

Those cases, and the hundreds of other heart patients I've cared for since my training as a cardiologist—much perspiration, indeed—leads me to describe what I call the thirty-year miracle. We have witnessed an amazing trajectory in the treatment of coronary artery disease over the past three decades.

✦ ✦ ✦

It was 1980 and I was a medical intern (physician-in-training) standing at the bedside of one of my patients in the intensive care unit. He was in the midst of a heart attack with severe chest pain, with significant changes on his cardiogram test, predictive of impending severe damage. I've got nothing to offer except pain medicine and nitroglycerin. Just that week my supervising resident physician had given me a new article from the medical literature about the use of long-acting nitrates like nitroglycerin in coronary artery disease. That's where we were. I was watching a man have a heart attack. I was perspiring but not because I was doing much.

✧ ✧ ✧

Now take a time-lapse journey with me ahead through the subsequent thirty years. New medicines (beta blockers and calcium channel blockers) were added to our armamentarium to protect the heart in the midst of a heart attack. Then a new study was published in a prestigious medical journal about *plaques* (deposits of cholesterol, fat, and calcium on artery walls) rupturing inside the coronary arteries and forming clots when a heart attack occurs. This was the inspiration we needed. This led to the era of clot-busting therapy and debates about the best way to break apart clots in the coronary arteries *before* permanent damage to heart muscle occurs—lots of perspiration trying to figure that out.

The whole thing was messy since this therapy affected the whole body—what breaks up dangerous clots in the heart arteries can cause dangerous bleeding elsewhere. That led to the question of whether we should try to deliver the clot-busting drugs directly into the heart arteries (rather than to the whole body) by *catheterization* (where a tube is inserted through a vein in the groin and threaded up into the heart) while the patient was in the midst of a heart attack. More perspiration that ultimately led us to conclude catheterization and squirting clot-busting medicines directly into the heart arteries is a good thing.

And then we had coronary *stents*. Stents are small pieces of mesh that are threaded into the arteries of the heart and used to stretch the narrowed or blocked arteries. Not great at first because of the high rate of clotting in the stents, causing the arteries to become blocked again. And it could take hours to deliver the stent into the artery. The technology was early, and better guidewires and steering devices were yet to come. Medicated stents to prevent re-blockage were the next big thing. They were much better and by now easier to deliver into the artery. There were still problems but lots of perspiration and bursts of technological inspiration led to better stents and anti-clotting treatments that reduced the re-blockage rate to a low level.

Which brings us to the twenty-first century. Dr. Eugene Braunwald has been at the forefront of cardiology for the past fifty years, providing much of the inspiration. He showed us that "Time is muscle." The faster we act, the less damage occurs to heart muscle during a heart attack. What can we do in the midst of a heart attack to help? We now know there is clot in the heart artery, and we have great stents to open blocked arteries, and we have better anti-clotting regimens to prevent re-blockage, and we know quick action is better. So we now take patients with certain types of heart attacks immediately to the catheterization room to get to the culprit artery as quickly as we can and put a stent in it. This process has been working so well that it is now done in local community hospitals without surgical backup. I wish I knew then what I know now. My patient back in 1980, having the heart attack while I could do little more than watch, would have called it a miracle.

It seems like it was medieval times when we were treating heart attacks thirty years ago. We may have done as much good by throwing a few leeches on (actually leeches might have led to some clot-busting, but that's another story entirely). What will the next thirty years bring—or for that matter, the next thirty months, or thirty days? Our continued perspiration, with bursts of inspiration, is already leading us to improve stents further (making them biodegradable, for example), and trying to identify the vulnerable plaque that might rupture in a coronary artery *before* it happens.

An evolution over thirty years may not be what people generally refer to as a miracle, unless of course you are on the receiving end of an extraordinarily effective stent at the time of a heart attack and end up with no permanent damage to your heart. As I look back, as I suppose many of us do at this time in our careers, and see the transformation in what we can do and what might be coming down the road, it is nothing short of miraculous.

DATE OF EVENT: 1996

A Miracle in Its Day, and Then Another

Mark F. Cotton, MMed (Paed), PhD

The setting is Cape Town, South Africa, in early 1996. Although we were seeing increasing numbers of cases of babies born with AIDS, there were no public programs in place yet for treating or preventing the infection in babies. Today, of course, we have effective medicines for both mothers and babies with the infection, but twenty years ago there were no medicines available in the public sector (the few wealthy patients with AIDS could purchase medicines privately). Today we have effective programs to prevent transmission of HIV from infected mothers to their babies—then we had no such programs. Today we have special clinics for HIV-infected adults, children, and babies—there were essentially none in 1996, and at the time we didn't even realize the extent of the problem. We hadn't started documenting the cases yet because they were difficult to recognize and the tests to make the diagnosis were either not widely available or of little utility—it did no good to know about an infection we could do nothing about.

So babies came to our clinic or were admitted to our hospital with the ravages of AIDS, and there was nothing to offer them. These are the stories of two babies with AIDS, very early in the South African epidemic of the disease, when we were happy to take any small miracles we could get.

CASE ONE

A nine-month-old boy was admitted to our hospital with severe block-age of his upper airway. This means that he was not able to adequately move air from his nose and throat into his lungs. The cause of his obstruction was extreme enlargement of his tonsils and adenoids, and swollen lymph nodes protruding into the back of his throat. We initially treated him with medi-cines to relieve his symptoms, such as decongestants, and a spray of steroids into his nose to reduce the inflammation. We gave him continuous oxygen through a tube that went from his nose to the back of his throat. Because of several other worrisome findings on his physical examination, such as a yeast infection in his mouth (thrush), an enlarged liver and spleen, and severe weight loss, we tested him for AIDS. Not surprisingly, he was positive. He had his tonsils and adenoids taken out and his breathing improved enough to go home. Recall from my comments earlier, we were not yet treating kids with AIDS medicines in South Africa.

Unfortunately, four days after going home he came back to the hospital extremely ill with right-sided heart failure, caused by a recurrence of the profound obstruction in his upper airway. Again, we gave continuous oxygen supplementation through a tube in his nose, but whenever we tried to stop the oxygen, he deteriorated. We knew that without doing something dramatic, this child would die. The only remaining approach was to surgically bypass the obstruction in his nose and the back of his throat with a tracheostomy, a breathing tube placed through the skin of the neck directly into the windpipe.

A tracheostomy is a major procedure and a big step for any child. For this child with AIDS, it presented even greater challenges. In 1996, our knowledge and practice of precautions to prevent the transmission of AIDS to hospital workers were also in their early stages. Surgeons were not eager to operate on patients with AIDS, and nurses were not eager to care for AIDS patients with lots of secretions to handle. A patient with a tracheostomy will not only have a bloody surgical wound, but will also require frequent suctioning of respiratory secretions through the tube in his neck. Suctioning can result in sprays of secretions—in an AIDS patient, those secretions may be infectious. In those days, nurses and doctors weren't even routinely wearing protective eyewear and masks in the intensive care unit where this child would be cared for. And tracheostomy would only be a temporary solution at best—it would not reduce the upper airway obstruction, and would require prolonged hospitalization for management; he could not be sent home with a tracheostomy.

To quell the growing objections to performing the tracheostomy, we "negotiated" with the nurses to give the child a course of treatment with the first anti-AIDS drug developed, called AZT (*azidothymidine*). As noted earlier, we did not have the resources to treat patients with AIDS, but we did have some AZT on hand to protect healthcare workers from needle-stick injuries. We made the case to the nurses that AZT would decrease the amount of virus in the child's body, his blood, and his secretions, making handling him in surgery and afterward less risky for them. They agreed, and we began the child on AZT in anticipation of performing the tracheostomy procedure shortly thereafter. We had no expectation of a treatment effect of the AZT—we were hoping only to reduce the number of viruses in his body long enough to more safely do the surgery.

However, to our utter amazement, almost immediately after starting the AZT therapy the little boy's upper airway obstruction melted away. In fact, within a day, he was already much improved. We had never had an experience like this where a severe, life-threatening complication of AIDS disappeared with barely a "whiff" of medicines. The tracheostomy procedure was no longer necessary, his heart failure resolved, and the child went home three weeks later on AZT therapy. Because of how stunning his recovery had been, and arguing that even expensive medicine was cheaper than surgery, we were able to convince the hospital to provide the child with AZT at home for six months. That's how long therapy with a single anti-AIDS drug could be effective in adults. The hospital argued that providing expensive medicine for longer than six months would not improve the outcome. We saw the child twice in follow-up over the next four months and he looked well on both visits. After that, he didn't return for further scheduled visits.

We are not naïve enough to think he was permanently cured of his AIDS—that would be unheard of with only a short-term course of treatment with a single drug. We now know that we can repress the AIDS infection long-term with three simultaneously, and continuously, given effective anti-AIDS drugs. But for this child, on the doorstep of the operating room for a dangerous and controversial procedure, this dramatic improvement in the major symptom of his AIDS, the upper airway blockage, was a miracle. And, considering all the alternative worse outcomes we might have faced, we were thrilled to be able to make this little boy's life a little better.

As a sign of how early in the African history of childhood AIDS this "miracle" occurred, my colleagues and I published this case in the medical literature and it was the first ever documented case of treating a child with AZT in Africa. We subsequently tested a stored blood sample from the baby and found that he was also infected with EBV (*Epstein-Barr virus*), the virus that causes *mononucleosis* ("mono"). EBV infection is well known to cause enlarged tonsils, adenoids, and lymph nodes in children in the West, but it typically causes few symptoms in young kids, especially under a year of age. In this little boy, we concluded his AIDS infection made his EBV worse and caused his severe upper airway obstruction. By treating his AIDS infection with AZT, we allowed his body to control the EBV infection.

This miracle was thankfully just the beginning of the miracles with anti-AIDS medicines, as the next case illustrates.

CASE TWO

Shortly after our experience with the little boy described above, a little girl born with AIDS infection developed one of the most dread complications of that disease: long-term, unremitting diarrhea. She had been on our hospital ward for more than six months, unable to gain weight, and continuously dehydrated. She required hundreds of painful needle pokes for intravenous (IV) lines that failed, or became infected, or simply fell out during this lengthy hospital stay. She was wasting away, unable to absorb food due to the severe diarrhea. The more she wasted and became dehydrated, the more IVs she needed, the more painful needle pokes, and the longer the hospitalization. Chronic diarrhea in AIDS babies is a vicious cycle of suffering, often ending only with death.

I remember the mother of this child well. She was a lovely but very young woman, and a caring mother. She had AIDS and was, as is typical, the source of the baby's infection. The baby also had physical findings suggestive of fetal alcohol syndrome, the result of her mom's drinking during pregnancy. But neither the mother's drinking problem, nor her own AIDS, nor her teenage youth stopped her from being a great mom to her little girl. The young mom's own mother, the baby's grandmother, was the cornerstone of this family and very involved in both her daughter's and her granddaughter's care.

Because of our extraordinary experience with the earlier case, we convinced the hospital to allow us to treat this baby with AZT as well—arguing that anything that might allow this baby to go home would be a victory. Once again, as with the first case, this baby's response to AZT was dramatic and almost instantaneous. Her diarrhea stopped, she gained weight, she no longer needed IVs or supplementary fluids, and she was able to go home. Her mother and her grandmother, who never thought their baby would be home again, were overjoyed. They proclaimed this to be a miracle. I proclaimed it as such also. The AZT didn't cure her AIDS; in fact, she died several months later. But she died at home, without diarrhea, having had quality weeks with her family.

Today, this baby would not have been born infected. Her mother would have been diagnosed with AIDS during pregnancy, treated with anti-AIDS medicines, and given birth to a healthy little girl. In the event the baby was born with AIDS today, perhaps because her mother's diagnosis wasn't made in a timely fashion, the baby would have been treated early with triple therapy (three effective AIDS drugs given simultaneously), and never would have developed chronic, unremitting diarrhea. But that's today. In 1996, being able to send a child with AIDS home after six months in the hospital with diarrhea was a previously unknown possibility. Without the first case of the little boy described above, we never would have been able to treat this little girl.

Again, we were thrilled to have another miracle in its day.

Triple therapy for AIDS didn't become widely available in South Africa until 2004. Until then, as a result of the two "miracle" cases above, we successfully used therapy with a single drug as a stopgap measure in some of our toughest cases of childhood AIDS, reducing hospitalizations, reducing babies' suffering, and improving the quality of life for these children.

For more about using single drug anti-AIDS therapy in resource-poor countries:

M Pijnenburg, M Cotton. Monotherapy in an era of combination therapy: is there a benefit? Experience in HIV-1-infected symptomatic South African children. *Annals of Tropical Paediatrics* 2000; 20: 185–192.

DATE OF EVENT: EARLY 1990s

With a Little Help from My Friends

David Spiegel, MD

"I've had metastases to my brain three times," Sheila told her support group of women with advanced breast cancer. "And each time I knew God would heal me. And he did. My doctors said, 'You're a walking miracle, all three times." Sheila was indeed born again—in her faith, and, she was sure, through her faith. She took what anyone else would see as a terrifying defeat, a sign of serious progression of her relentless disease, and saw it as an opportunity for God to prove his love. She had been diagnosed with inflammatory breast cancer, a particularly aggressive type, at age thirty-two. Her breast went from acutely painful to completely discolored in three weeks. After consulting with a number of doctors, she elected not to have a mastectomy, but to have a full course of chemotherapy and radiation.

"I could tell from the way the young doctors looked at me, they thought: 'She's dead meat, don't get too attached. Use it as a learning experience.' The first night I had chemo, I got deathly ill. My husband was there. I turned to him and said, 'I can't do this.' I prayed to the Lord: 'Lord, if this is the way it's gonna be, just take me now.' I never vomited again, I never got sick again. After that I had a lot people praying, a lot of support, family, friends. I came through it with shining colors."

I had just started my career in academic psychiatry with an extraordinary opportunity. A highly regarded group psychotherapist and renowned author at my institution had invited me to co-lead a new support group he had assembled of women with *metastatic* (where cancer has spread to other sites in the body) breast cancer. He was writing a textbook on existential psychotherapy, and was interested in the concept that you don't really live authentically until you confront death, i.e., face the possibility of your own nonbeing. If that was true, as Kierkegaard, Sartre, and Heidegger had written, then perhaps dealing with life-threatening disease could be an occasion for growth, not decline. At the time, some oncologists thought we would demoralize these women by assembling them in a weekly support group. After all, the median survival with metastatic breast cancer then was just two years. The oncologists feared women in such groups would watch one another die, seeing the worst, not extracting the best from the experience.

But to the contrary, we found the women in our groups formed strong bonds with one another, coming to see in each other what they had more trouble seeing in themselves: their courage and resoluteness in the face of punishing treatments and advancing disease. They came to feel like experts in living, giving one another advice about everything from getting test results early, to what to tell friends and family. And they learned to stare death in the eye.

As one group member put it, "Being in the group is like looking into the Grand Canyon when you are afraid of heights. You know it would be a disaster if you fell, but you feel better about yourself because you're able to look. That is how I feel about death in the group. I can't say I feel serene, but I can look at it."

Sheila told the group, "My main objective was to help someone else regain hope, because you can get through it." At the first meeting after a member of the group died unexpectedly, Sheila said with tears in her eyes, "I invested in her, I had feelings for her. I wish I could talk to her."

When I asked her, "What would you say to her?"

Sheila said, "Not to worry. Not to fear. To have somebody there to tell you that, and that it's okay, your family will be all right, and not to feel guilty for being sick, for dying on them. They will be okay—they will continue." As she spoke, she was comforting the other members of the group in their grief for our lost member, and, of course, in their thoughts about their own mortality.

Sheila seemed so certain. She was there to help others, and she showed so little concern about her own dire situation that it made me uncomfortable. Was it denial, a defense against existential terror? I was there to help these women using a psychotherapy that sought to guide them in expressing all the emotions associated with advancing cancer: anger, fear, and sadness, as well as to use those feelings to savor the sweetness of life and relationships, and to find meaning in whatever time we all had left. Was Sheila short-circuiting this process with her serene belief? Nothing ruffled her conviction, even another group member's none-too-conciliatory statement that "I don't believe there is any intelligence in this universe that cares one bit what happens to any of us."

Sheila later commented, "She was a downright atheist—in my face all the time—she almost ran me out of the room. She had a very strong personality. I almost let her do that to me, but I realized that wasn't my purpose. My purpose was to stay. That was the whole purpose of the group—to express our feelings."

In order to see whether we were indeed demoralizing the women in our groups, we assessed the content of the group's discussions in relation to the prevailing emotions minute-by-minute. We found that the specter of death powerfully influenced the depth of our discussions, but did not lead to an over-whelming negative mood. Indeed, we found that the more open the women were about all emotions, the more their anxiety and depression *decreased* over time, rather than increased. Sheila could talk about death, but didn't seem to worry about it. Compared to other women in the group, who had metastases to their bones, which is painful, her condition was worse: the tumors had appeared in her brain. Yet she showed no sign of mental impairment, came weekly to the group, and her spirits were high. She was there to "help others."

Our group was part of a National Institutes of Health-funded study designed to re-evaluate the effects of group psychotherapy. In an earlier study we had recruited eighty-six women in all, and randomly (equivalent to the toss of a coin) assigned fifty of them to weekly support groups; the other thirty-six received their standard medical care without special emotional support. We followed them all over many years, and found that the women in our support program were better off emotionally, and had less pain as well. We taught them self-hypnosis for that.

I got curious about one more outcome measure—how long these women survived. We had begun the project in the late 1970s, when books were being written about *imaging* away your cancer by picturing your white blood cells killing your cancer cells, and how people got cancer because of some deep emotional "need" for it. I felt this was blaming the victim, and that there was no evidence that such mental imagery or painful introspection could affect the course of cancer. In any event, we were doing the opposite in our groups: facing death and detoxifying the fear, not wishing the disease away. So in the late 1980s I obtained death records for all of the women in our study. Not surprisingly, by then eighty-three of the eighty-six had died. But what was astonishing to me was the fact that, on average, the women assigned to our support groups lived eighteen months longer than the controls who had not received special emotional support, while receiving the same type and quantity of medical treatment. By four years after the study had begun, all of the control patients had died, while one-third of the women in group therapy were still alive.

We published that finding in a leading medical journal in 1989. Since then, eight of fifteen published randomized clinical trials have shown that psychotherapeutic support results in longer cancer survival, while the other seven show no difference. None of the studies show that talking about death *shortens* life. We did another study involving 125 women beginning in 1990 to confirm our results. Although we did not find a survival advantage for *all* of the women in the new study, we did find the same group therapy benefit on survival in those women with tumors that didn't respond to hormone therapy. Breast cancer therapy had improved considerably over the fifteen years since our original study, especially hormonal treatments, making it harder to demonstrate the improved survival effect of group psychotherapy. But in those women who didn't benefit from the newer hormonal therapy, group psychotherapy could still be shown to improve survival. Indeed, an authoritative review in 2013 of all the literature in the field concluded that group therapy improves survival with breast cancer.

The power of social support is further demonstrated by a recent population study involving 734,889 cancer patients showing that simply being married is associated with four months' longer survival, equivalent to the effect of many kinds of chemotherapy. So living better also means living longer.

Sheila's faith was not misplaced. As she put it, "If I hadn't had faith, I would have gone nuts. If I hadn't had faith, I would have committed suicide. Looking back, my cancer was a blessing because it allowed me to reevaluate my life, what was important, who was important, get rid of all the deadwood relationships that were not sincere. With a disease like that your real friends hang in there, and the ones that were not with you are gone. I feel I am in the protective circle of his love. It doesn't mean I don't get depressed, but at the end of the tunnel, I'm okay. Look into his light, not to the left or the right, don't get distracted by things that are hurtful."

While she is no longer with us, Sheila lived for *twenty-four years* after she joined the group, while the average survival time for women in the study was two and a half years. Just as she predicted to the others in her group years before, her family is okay. So are we, for having known her.

For more information on our studies of group therapy's impact on breast cancer survival, see:

Spiegel, D., J. R. Bloom, H. C. Kraemer and E. Gottheil (1989). "Effect of psychosocial treatment on survival of patients with metastatic breast cancer." *Lancet* 2(8668): 888–891.

Spiegel, D., L. D. Butler, J. Giese-Davis, C. Koopman, E. Miller, S. DiMiceli, C. C. Classen, P. Fobair, R. W. Carlson and H. C. Kraemer (2007). "Effects of supportive-expressive group therapy on survival of patients with metastatic breast cancer: a randomized prospective trial." *Cancer* 110(5): 1130–1138.

Spiegel, D. (2011). "Mind matters in cancer survival." *JAMA* 305(5): 502–503.

For more on existential psychotherapy, see:

Yalom, I. D. (1980). *Existential Psychotherapy.* New York, Basic Books.

Yalom, I. D. (2008). Staring at the Sun: Overcoming the Terror of Death. San Francisco, Jossey-Bass

For an extensive review of the literature on group therapy's impact on breast cancer survival, see:

Mustafa, M., A. Carson-Stevens, D. Gillespie and A. G. Edwards (2013). "Psychological interventions for women with metastatic breast cancer." Cochrane Database Syst Rev 6: CD004253.

For more information on the benefit of marriage on cancer survival, see:

Aizer, A. A., M. H. Chen, E. P. McCarthy, M. L. Mendu, S. Koo, T. J. Wilhite, P. L. Graham, T. K. Choueiri, K. E. Hoffman, N. E. Martin, J. C. Hu and P. L. Nguyen (2013). "Marital status and survival in patients with cancer." *Journal of Clinical Oncology* 31(31): 3869–3876.

9

Paying It Forward

Patients and families, grateful for the miracles they've received, may seek to channel that gratitude into meaningful action on behalf of others. Those actions can have dramatic impacts and help create miracles of the future. Three of the essays in this chapter describe such phenomena—the amplification of one miraculous outcome to create many more.

Two other essays describe young people, the beneficiaries of medical miracles in their own lives, who were then inspired to pursue medical careers that have benefitted countless others.

DATE OF EVENT: 1995

Sharing the Miracle of Hope

Trevor J. Bayliss, MD

I never thought I'd end up being a doctor. I never even thought I'd survive long enough to graduate college. But today I am an oncologist, a physician specializing in the treatment of patients with cancer. Twenty years ago, I was a college freshman diagnosed with terminal cancer, given only weeks or, at most, months to live. My survival was a miracle, for which I'm grateful every day. This is my story.

✧ ✧ ✧

I had been a star runner and ice hockey player in high school. Competing in those sports had become a passion and a part of my identity, and when I enrolled at Williams College I had plans to continue my athletics. But as soon as I began training with the cross-country team in the fall of my freshman year in 1994, I knew something wasn't right: I was too easily fatigued, couldn't maintain the times I had run in high school. The same thing happened when I tried to play hockey that winter. I was exhausted, no energy, and felt drained after every practice.

In the spring when I went out for track and field, I also noticed my abdomen was getting bigger. Others noticed, too. During a swimming pool workout with the track team, my coach called out, "You look like you're pregnant, Bayliss." Indeed, I did look pregnant, but it turned out the growth inside of me was my spleen, which had enlarged to massive proportions. The spleen is the organ in our body that filters our blood; when it gets clogged, it swells.

In the summer of 1995 a thorough medical evaluation discovered I had a rare (fewer than 100 cases each year in the United States) form of blood cancer, called *T-cell LGL* (for large granular lymphocytic) leukemia. I had surgery to take out my spleen, which the doctors said would make me feel better immediately, and it did. The surgeon told me it was the largest spleen he had ever removed, which for a naturally competitive guy like me, gave me a somewhat perverse sense of achievement. The extreme fatigue I had been feeling, the doctors explained, was surely due to the anemia caused by my blood cells being trapped in my enormous spleen, unable to filter through because of the leukemia cells that were clogging it.

Because most cases of this type of leukemia are very "indolent," or slow-growing, my doctors didn't feel I needed additional therapy at that time, in hopes the leukemia cells would remain dormant. I was put on a "watch and wait" plan, which was a difficult concept—knowing I had cancer inside of me, but doing nothing about it. Things continued okay through my sophomore year of college; it seemed I did have the usual indolent version of this leukemia. Although unable to participate in sports, I was feeling well overall. Yet I was always anxious about the idea of this disease lurking inside of me.

As my junior year of college began, friends began commenting that my lips looked a little bluish. One day I climbed half a flight of stairs in my dorm and found myself hunched over trying to regain my breath. I was startled by that event and went back to my doctor, who saw suspicious shadows on my chest X-ray, confirmed abnormalities on a chest CAT scan (a special type of X-ray), and suggested a lung biopsy. The biopsy found the leukemia had infiltrated my lungs and, by so doing, declared itself to no longer be "indolent." Further testing found leukemia cells in my liver as well. "Watch and wait" would no longer be sufficient.

Unfortunately, my version of T-cell LGL turned out to be unusual in a number of ways, not the least of which was that it usually occurred in sixty-year-olds, and I was nineteen when I was diagnosed. But much worse, although T-cell LGL usually is either aggressive from the beginning or indolent throughout its course, tests showed that what was initially behaving as an indolent leukemia in me had transitioned to the aggressive form seemingly overnight. My oncologist said I needed to start chemotherapy immediately, a combination of four drugs that I tolerated pretty well except for a day of fever, predictable with each cycle of treatment, and some general fatigue. I didn't have to be hospitalized for the therapy and I was still able to attend a couple classes during November and December of my junior year. But the cancer didn't disappear on this chemotherapy protocol, and my doctors said a bone marrow transplant was my only hope of surviving this now-aggressive form of T-cell LGL.

I traveled with my mom to a famous cancer and bone marrow transplant center on the West Coast where I would receive the transplant. Bone marrow transplant replaces a patient's bone marrow (where blood cells are made, and this type of cancer resides) with an infusion of bone marrow stem cells from a matched donor. Although I didn't have a match in my family, the National Bone Marrow Registry located a match from an anonymous donor. Bone marrow transplant is a dangerous procedure for many reasons. Before the transplant, the patient has to have very intensive rounds of chemotherapy, much harsher than what I had received before, in an attempt to wipe out every cancer cell before the transplant. The chemotherapy also wipes out a lot of normal cells. I went through this treatment and became very debilitated, physically and emotionally. Following the intense chemotherapy, a patient must then have whole body radiation to wipe out his immune system so his own body won't reject the transplanted bone marrow. Without an immune system, a patient is prone to serious infections. Finally, after the transplant, the new bone marrow itself can attack the patient's body, something called *graft-versus-host disease*.

Following my chemotherapy, though, all of those concerns about the additional dangers of the upcoming bone marrow transplant became moot. A meeting was called one week before the scheduled transplant with me, my mom, the oncologist at the cancer center, and a nurse. The oncologist entered the room quietly and sat across the table from me. I could quickly tell by her awkward manner and the uncomfortable look on her face that this was not going to proceed according to plan. Something had happened. My cancer had not responded well even to the intense chemotherapy of the past weeks; it was now advancing in my lungs, reducing the amount of oxygen in my system. I needed to receive supplemental oxygen from a tube in my nose hooked up to a portable oxygen tank. And then the final blow: because of these new developments and the results of the latest round of tests, there was now a 95 percent chance the bone marrow transplant procedure, if performed, would fail and perhaps even kill me. There were no good options left. After a painful silence in the room, I asked the question cancer patients given terminal diagnoses often ask: "How long do I have?"

The oncologist's answer: "Months, maybe only weeks." As I absorbed the words I felt a lump forming in my throat, tears welling in my eyes, and I knew I had about three words I could get out without completely breaking down. I turned to my mom, who was obviously devastated by the news, and said, "Let's go home."

The night after my meeting with the doctor I lay in bed crying, for the first time accepting that I may die very soon. As I did, I surprisingly felt a peace come over me, a lifting of the fear. And just as quickly I found myself planning for the future. Initially it was only the immediate future of getting home and seeing my family and friends. As I flew home two days later, at 30,000 feet wearing oxygen, I replayed in my head that last meeting at the cancer center. I realized how hard it must have been for the doctor to say what she had to say, but at the same time, I found myself thinking, *I could do that well. I could do that better, and with more compassion, than that doctor had done.* As sick as I was, leaving there with no hope, that was the first inkling I had that I wanted to be a doctor, I wanted to help people with cancer. How impossible, even delusional, that felt at the time.

The oncologist's answer to my "how long" was what we now call "evidence-based," meaning that it comes from careful analysis of scientific data from published medical literature and from doctors' own experience with their patients. It's an average, a bell-shaped curve. At the middle of the curve, patients in my situation survived weeks to months, just as the doctor had said. But there was something about how the oncologist said it that disturbed me; I was not a statistic. There must be factors that determine which patients live longer than the average, and which live shorter than the average. As I wrote in the *Dartmouth Medicine* magazine several years later:

> Perhaps it's the biology of their cancer cells, or perhaps certain personality or attitude traits. I tended to hold to the latter view and believed that if I faced my illness forthrightly, meditated, visualized, and fought, I'd be among those who lived longer than average.
>
> Some doctors stayed away from statistics, and I preferred that even more. The ones who used statistics wanted to place me right on the average and test my hope at each appointment. I understood that it was their duty to let patients know what they faced. I was even able to admit that my hope at times bordered on denial. But denial and hope are closely linked and, I think, often blur together.
>
> *Dartmouth Medicine* Summer 2010

I returned without having the transplant that was supposed to have saved my life, the procedure that had been my only hope. I was going home to die. But, surrounded by family and friends, I couldn't imagine dying. Throughout this ordeal, as serious as I knew my cancer was, I had never really confronted the possibility of death before. Sure, I had broken down and cried a couple of times, and in the back of my mind I knew things may go badly. But how could I die in my twenties? I really didn't feel that badly; recovering from the assault of the chemotherapy, I seemed to be getting a little of my strength back. I knew I still had a runner's healthy heart going for me. I saw my hometown oncologist and he agreed that I looked pretty good for a dying man. "You don't look that sick." I can't tell you how important hearing that from him was to me, even if it was only meant to temporarily cheer me up. It was exactly what I needed to hear—and it was exactly how I felt. I didn't feel like I was on death's door. Indeed, "denial and hope are closely linked and often blur together."

My hometown oncologist had spoken with an international expert in my rare cancer and had learned about a few patients with my type of cancer who had promising results with an experimental therapy using a medicine called *methotrexate*. In those few patients, the medicine had been given in relatively low doses and was well-tolerated. Methotrexate had been used for many years in patients with other conditions, including other types of cancers, but had never been studied in T-cell LGL. With nothing to lose, we decided to give it a try.

The results were dramatic. Within weeks I no longer needed my oxygen tube and tank, my blood counts were normalizing, and within a couple months there were almost no remaining leukemia cells in my blood. I went into a deep remission. To this day, seventeen years later, LGL leukemic cells can be found in my blood when viewed carefully under the microscope, but they are held in check.

My experience with my own cancer, and with the oncologist at the famous cancer center where I was told there was nothing more they could do for me, led me to my career as an oncologist. I graduated from Williams, actually competing at the NCAA National Championships as a senior on the track team. Just being on the track, able to breathe hard, able to breathe at all, was a victory. Winning the races I did was an unexpected bonus. I went on to Albany Medical College, and then did a residency and fellowship at Dartmouth-Hitchcock Medical Center in New Hampshire.

I am back to running for fun and in 5K and 10K races and have done a few marathons. My wife and I have three wonderful, beautiful sons. As an oncologist, I now care for patients with the whole spectrum of cancers; some of my patients are as young as I was when I was diagnosed. Every one of my patients pulls me back to my own experience, guiding me in how I speak to them and how I treat them. In a newspaper interview not too long ago, I said:

> I think the biggest thing I took from my experience and try to apply to others is honoring their story and just trying to listen. When you listen that way and want to get to know who they are, I want to know how they feel when they heard they have cancer. If you enter each encounter from that mindset and remembering what it was like for me at each of those steps, to hear I have cancer, to hear I have no more options and being able to check back to that moment and think about it as I go into a room with a patient in invaluable.
>
> *USA Today*, May 15, 2014

I see each day of my life as a gift, a miracle, and I try to help my patients see their lives that way as well. I know all too well how difficult that can be when in the throes of serious illness and receiving difficult treatments, but it's become my personal mission in life.

To read the complete *Dartmouth Medicine* piece:

http://dartmed.dartmouth.edu/summer10/html/both_sides_now.php

To read the complete *USA Today* interview:

http://ftw.usatoday.com/2014/05/trevor-bayliss-williams-track-cancer-doctor-tbt

For more information about the National Bone Marrow Transplant Registry: *https://bethematch.org/*

DATE OF EVENT: 2001–2003

A Disappearing Tumor Becomes a Source of Hope for Many

Bradley A. George, MD

While he was still in the womb, Brandon's routine pregnancy ultrasound test showed a mass around his spinal cord. When Brandon was born, although the tumor was not visible from the outside, an MRI scan (magnetic resonance imaging is a way to see inside the body without using radiation) confirmed his parents' worst fears: there was a mass around his lower spine that extended between the vertebrae (spinal column bones) into the spinal canal where the nerve roots run.

We explained to Brandon's parents that this was most likely a rare childhood cancer called *neuroblastoma*, which originates in nerve cells. There are fewer than 1,000 cases of neuroblastoma diagnosed in the United States each year, and almost all of them occur in very young children. This can be a very aggressive, dangerous, and even lethal tumor, but as some kids get older, these tumors sometimes actually shrink or go away entirely. It isn't possible to say with certainty which neuroblastomas will grow and spread and which will shrink or even disappear. Because of Brandon's age and the location and appearance of the tumor, we felt Brandon's neuroblastoma fit the category of tumor that had a good chance of spontaneously disappearing or "maturing" into a tumor that would no longer have malignant potential. He was additionally fortunate that the location of the tumor was at the lowest part of his spinal canal, beneath where the spinal cord ended, and therefore he was unlikely to have any problems with movement or bodily functions unless the tumor grew.

We recommended keeping a close eye on the tumor, holding off on surgery until we could determine whether it would grow or shrink. We explained that surgery in the spinal canal can itself be quite risky and could cause problems with nerve function, in addition to the risks associated with any surgery and anesthesia in a young baby—we felt careful observation was the best course for the time being. This is a difficult recommendation for any parent to accept. They know there's a neuroblastoma tumor in their baby, they've read all about neuroblastomas, and they know these tumors can be very dangerous, even life-threatening, often requiring surgery, chemotherapy, and/or radiation. And although our past experience with cases like this, as well as published studies from other cancer experts, predicted a favorable outcome for Brandon's tumor, we couldn't offer a guarantee that the tumor wouldn't grow or spread. If surgery was done now and there were no complications, Brandon might well be cured and not require any additional treatments. But, if we waited and watched, he might "cure himself," sparing him the risks of surgery.

Brandon's parents agreed, with understandable nervousness, to careful observation. Because the tumor wasn't visible on the outside, we followed him with frequent MRI scans. The tumor appeared perhaps to be very gradually shrinking; at least we could reassure Brandon's parents that the tumor wasn't growing or spreading. But it wasn't gone by any means. They knew there was still a potentially dangerous tumor inside their child's body. Added to that was the fact that although Brandon seemed fine, there was nothing they could "watch" from the outside for reassurance on a day-to-day basis, and we didn't have biopsy results to assess the exact type of tumor and "stage" of tumor we were dealing with—biopsy of a tumor in that proximity to the spine can itself be very hazardous.

When Brandon was eighteen months of age, we performed another MRI confirming the tumor was still there. At twenty-three months of age, in August 2003, Brandon developed fever and some bone pain, so we again repeated the MRI to make sure the symptoms weren't due to tumor progression, but the tumor was still stable. At that point, Brandon's parents began exploring the options for surgery. They contacted the excellent neurosurgery group at a major West Coast university medical center and arranged for Brandon to be assessed there for possible biopsy and surgery. Their first visit was in late August 2003. An MRI at that time again revealed a stable tumor. Brandon's parents arranged for him to return to the West Coast university medical center in November 2003 for biopsy and/or surgery.

When they arrived in November, three months after the most recent unchanged MRI, and two years after the tumor was first diagnosed, Brandon had another MRI to help guide the surgeons for the procedure scheduled for the next day. The results stunned Brandon's family and their doctors on the West Coast, who had reviewed all the previous scans and were preparing for surgery: the tumor was entirely gone, almost as if it disappeared mid-air on the flight from Atlanta.

Brandon's parents considered this a miracle and, certainly, the timing of the tumor's disappearance was remarkable and very fortuitous—just in the nick of time to spare the child the substantial risks of this type of surgery. But for those of us who had cared for Brandon in Atlanta, the miracles were just starting.

Brandon's mom, Kristin, was a corporate attorney for a big law firm in town. She had spent the previous eighteen months in and out of our children's oncology clinic waiting room, seeing all the kids who, like Brandon, had cancer. All types of cancer, few if any of which would "disappear" on their own. She met parents struggling with dire prognoses for their kids. Many of the kids playing with Brandon in the waiting area already had the severe telltale signs of chemotherapy or radiation or both. Others had undergone surgery or were about to.

Having a child escape the potential ravages of cancer and its treatment is more than enough to make any parent overjoyed and grateful. But, whereas most parents in that blessed situation would walk out of the oncology clinic with the relief of never having to confront those difficult days again, Kristin walked out of our clinic with a mission. First, she asked if she could help with fundraising for our program, which she did. A year following Brandon's visit to the West Coast medical center, Kristin took a leave of absence from her law practice to become the Senior Vice President of Community and Business Development at a national childhood cancer nonprofit. She also became involved with a small, local charitable organization called Cure Children's Cancer (CURE) that helped provide support for families of area kids with the disease. Following her early volunteer days with CURE, Kristin's efforts became all-consuming. She never returned to her law firm, instead dedicating her life to helping find a cure for kids with cancer.

Three years after Brandon's family's momentous trip to the West Coast medical center, Kristin became the Executive Director of CURE, a position she has now held for nearly ten years. In that time, this small, local organization has become a national force in fundraising for children's cancer care and research, raising millions of dollars each year. These desperately needed funds support our work with all types of cancer at our institution, but also support children's cancer programs across the country. CURE also maintains its original goal of supporting families as they go through the difficult journey with their children. The CURE mission statement and vision statement summarize the organization well:

> CURE Childhood Cancer is dedicated to conquering childhood cancer through funding targeted research and through support of patients and their families. CURE Childhood Cancer believes that childhood cancer can be cured in our lifetime.

Besides having had the privilege of caring for Brandon and other kids with cancer who now benefit by Kristin's work, I have another, very personal connection to Kristin and CURE. My oldest son and a friend of his started an annual fundraising run in the name of a young man, Sam, who went to the same high school as our son. Sam was a promising athlete who tragically died of metastatic bone cancer. All four of my children have been involved with organizing the run over the past eight years. The funds raised from the run go to the Sam Robb Fund of CURE. This fund, with the help and guidance of Sam's family and CURE, provides funds to support families going through their kids' cancer therapy, and also provides full funding for a fellowship in pediatric oncology at Children's Healthcare of Atlanta and Emory University. These fellows complete their clinical and research training with us and then join the world of children's cancer-fighting doctors.

Brandon's disappearing tumor was a miracle for his family. His mother's work since that time has been a miracle for all of us treating kids with cancer.

For more about CURE:

http://www.curechildhoodcancer.org/#sthash.i786wfd7.dpbs

For more about the CURE Sam Robb Fund:

http://www.curechildhoodcancer.org/named-funds/cure-named-funds/the-sam-robb-fund/#sthash .TLPbSnBY.dpbs

---

DATE OF EVENT: SUMMER 1993

Helping Create Miracles for Babies of the Future

Richard F. Jacobs, MD

As a clinical researcher, I test potential new therapies for children that may or may not ultimately be proven to be beneficial. This usually requires randomly assigning some children to a group receiving the experimental therapy and others to a group receiving the existing, standard treatment. If there is no existing therapy, the experimental group is compared with a group receiving a placebo ("sugar pill"). The outcomes of the groups are then studied to determine if the new therapy was safe and effective compared with previous therapies or, if there are no existing therapies, compared to no therapy at all. Before any patient can be included in a research study, they must be thoroughly educated about the study, including all the potential risks. The patient (or parents, in the case of a young child) must then formally agree to participate in the research study. That process is called obtaining *informed consent.*

It has always amazed me how willing, and even eager, parents are to help us seek new preventions, treatments, and cures for children, not knowing if the research study we are asking them to consider will benefit their own child. In 1993, we were conducting a very important research study, as part of a National Institutes of Health research network, of a medicine to treat babies infected at birth with a dangerous virus called cytomegalovirus or CMV. It was long known that babies who contracted a brain infection with CMV had a high likelihood of permanent and often total deafness. This particular research study required insertion of a deeply placed IV catheter (tube placed in a vein) to give an experimental medicine for six weeks to fight the CMV virus. The medicine was known to be effective in adults with various types of CMV infections, and its side effects were also well known in adults. But the medicine had never been studied in babies over such a long treatment period.

In this study, babies were to be randomly assigned to either have the deep IV catheter inserted and receive six weeks of treatment with the medicine, or be assigned to a "no treatment" control group, which would receive no IV catheter and no treatment. Because the deep IV catheter carries its own risks, it could not ethically be inserted into babies merely to give a placebo. As a result, unlike many studies where the doctors, patients, and families are all *unaware* of which patients are receiving an experimental medicine and which patients are not, in this study everyone would know because the "no treatment" patients would not even have the deep IV catheter inserted. This meant explaining to parents, while obtaining informed consent, that their baby would be randomly assigned to either receive the research medication we wanted to evaluate for possible benefit or, because there was no standard treatment available for CMV infection, their baby would receive no treatment at all. Although all babies in the study, whether receiving the experimental medicine or not, would be given a very comprehensive follow-up, testing, and a detailed assessment of all potential outcomes, parents would immediately know if their baby did or did not receive therapy.

Obtaining informed consent from parents requires conscientiously providing all information and as complete a description as possible so they can make a truly informed decision regarding what's best for their child. This great responsibility has always been an emotionally exhausting exercise for me. That is, until I met this particular family who made the process incredibly easy. I was explaining the CMV treatment study to them because their baby had CMV infection of the brain and was at high risk for deafness. Of course, as with all families, they wanted a treatment to help their baby and they asked complete and direct questions. But they started by saying they just wanted to help us answer the important medical questions we were addressing with the study, even if their baby was not one of those randomly assigned to receive the potentially beneficial medicine.

As it turned out, their son was randomly assigned to receive the experimental treatment and tolerated it well despite some challenges due to the side effect of depressed white blood cell counts, something we knew to expect from this research medication. When enough patients had been enrolled in the study and all the results were analyzed, the study did show that the experimental treatment was effective in decreasing hearing loss and preserving babies' hearing over time compared with the no-treatment group.

This wonderful family's son retained functional but somewhat decreased hearing, and the family opted to have cochlear implants inserted to bring their son's hearing up to completely normal levels. Every time I see his family, they hug me and tell me they are so happy to have helped prevent hearing loss for other babies like their son. The study was published in one of the leading pediatrics journals, and the parents even asked me for an autographed copy. While they are convinced the experimental medicine preserved enough hearing for their baby to be completely normalized subsequently by the cochlear implants, they are even more convinced of the benefits of today's research for children in the future. This medicine and another newer medicine based on it have continued to show promise in reducing deafness in CMV-infected babies, and they also appear to possibly reduce other ill effects of the infection in babies, including developmental delay and brain damage.

I am constantly invigorated by the human spirit of those wanting to help answer questions for the benefit of future patients.

DATE OF EVENT:1975

Making Miracles for Others

Celia I. Kaye, MD, PhD

I was providing consultations at a community hospital as a newly trained geneticist, a specialist in diagnosing and treating inherited diseases. Sarah was just a few months old, with severe, ongoing, and long-lasting diarrhea that had required hospitalization and IV fluids (given directly into a vein) for several weeks of her short life. Although we didn't know what her diagnosis was, we did know she was failing. It was generally agreed that she was too small and fragile to survive, but we were still desperately trying to save her. Our goal was to keep her alive long enough to determine what was wrong with her in hopes that knowledge would lead to her treatment and cure. She was the first child to her young parents, who were terrified they might lose their baby and frustrated by our inability to help her. Since this was before the days we had the capability of giving adequate nutrition intravenously, Sarah was starving to death before our eyes.

Sarah had a range of problems outside of my experience. As a very young and relatively inexperienced "expert," I was at a loss to figure out what was wrong with her. Doing what others in my position routinely do, I sought help from colleagues elsewhere and found many who, despite not even knowing this patient, gave of their time and energy to help from a distance. After talking to gastroenterology specialists (physicians treating stomach and intestinal disorders) and other genetics experts, we decided to try Sarah on a very new and still unproven type of baby formula that contained only the basic building blocks of nutrients rather than the complex nutrients found in standard baby formulas. We didn't feel we had a choice—it was clear this baby would die if we continued standard formulas. It was a long and difficult trial, but Sarah ultimately was able to tolerate the new formula, gained weight, and was able to go home with her parents, much to their relief and ours.

This was only the first step of a long odyssey of trying to figure out what was wrong with Sarah, prompted by the emergence of many new problems as the years passed. Although her intellectual development was normal and she met her childhood milestones, Sarah always had difficulty with feedings and diet, and her growth was very slow. She developed unusual skin changes. In later years, an abnormality in her bone marrow occurred, resulting in not enough mature blood cells circulating in her body, perplexing the blood and bone marrow experts. Despite these many complications, Sarah continued to progress well in other ways, went to school, and ultimately on to college. She was always the "different one," requiring lots of medical attention, missing school, looking smaller and frailer than her friends. Sarah's parents never wavered in their love and support for her, despite the ongoing emergence of new medical troubles that always seemed to surprise the experts. Now Sarah is in her thirties, and I have still never learned the cause of her illness, and her future remains uncertain.

Although close to death when I first saw her, she "hung on" until we were able to find a way to feed her. Against all odds and all the experts' predictions, Sarah lived. Of course, to her parents and to those of us taking care of her, this was a miracle. But perhaps an even greater miracle is how Sarah has responded to her numerous life-threatening medical developments and ongoing medical challenges.

Sarah has chosen a career helping children find their own normalcy when faced with chronic medical problems—problems, like hers, that never go away. She has had the energy and the courage to turn her own story into one that can help others, and she is doing this every day. She is determined to make the future brighter for other children who will always be different from their friends and classmates. For those kids, Sarah is now a miracle maker.

DATE OF EVENT: 1956

A Dramatic Cure Leads to Many More

Michael S. Kappy, MD

Harley A. Rotbart, MD

Mike was a sixteen-year-old boy who had experienced a week of increasing numbness and weakness that was gradually ascending up his body from his feet toward his head. There are several very serious conditions that can cause these symptoms, including polio, lead poisoning, and a paralytic neurological condition called Guillain-Barré syndrome (GBS). He was admitted to a large community hospital over fifty years ago and treated emergently with injections of "British anti-Lewisite," a medicine that was developed back in World War II to treat arsenic poisoning from chemical warfare. The same medicine was effective in other heavy metal poisonings like lead, and lead poisoning was one of the possibilities in this case. But, after many rounds of tests, Mike was ultimately determined to have GBS.

Mike went on to develop all of the dreaded complications of GBS, including paralysis and failure of the part of his nervous system that controls breathing. Early one morning, he suddenly went into cardiorespiratory arrest—his breathing and heart stopped. After a prolonged and difficult resuscitation, and the recognition that he could not breathe on his own, Mike was placed in an *iron lung* machine, named such because iron lungs were made of metal and could help a patient to breathe.

Iron lung machines are now obsolete because we have modern *ventilator* machines (also caused *positive pressure ventilators*) that can *actively* pump air into and out of patients' lungs when their own breathing fails. But before positive pressure ventilator machines were developed, the only way to move air through the lungs of paralyzed patients was *passively*, using the iron lung (also called *negative pressure ventilator*). The iron lung is a body-size metal tube connected to a vacuum pump. The patient is placed inside the tube, which forms a seal around the patient's body. The machine cycles through suction and non-suction phases, the pace of which can be controlled by the doctors. When the suction part of the cycle was on, the iron lung would expand the patient's chest cavity, drawing air into the lungs; when the suction was turned off, the chest cavity would return to its resting state, expelling the air. Only the patient's head extended outside the machine. Mike remembers being told that if he had been an inch taller, he wouldn't have fit! There were no breathing tubes involved as there are now with ventilator machines that directly deliver air into the lungs. The machine functioned a little like a mouth on a straw, and the body was the straw—when suction was applied, air entered Mike's lungs, and when suction was released, air was released. Iron lung machines were widely used to treat the most severe forms of polio, in which patients' breathing muscles were paralyzed, often permanently.

The doctors treating Mike were desperately hoping that the successful resuscitation and breathing support he was receiving would allow him to recover, since most, but by no means all, patients with GBS slowly regain their muscle function.

Indeed, Mike gradually regained his ability to move and breathe over a three-week period, and he was then treated with physical therapy for several months, including a three-month stay in a physical medicine rehabilitation hospital. Over the ensuing several months, he regained nearly all of his movement functions. Mike went on to graduate from high school. The path he then chose for his career, after surviving his life-threatening illness and witnessing the heroic efforts his caregivers made to pull him through, is a remarkable example of giving back, and it illustrates how miracles can ensue from "paying it forward."

Mike went on to college and then to medical school. During his residency training, he helped establish a free clinic in a depressed and underserved neighborhood in Washington, DC. Following his residency, he established an urban clinic in another underserved city, providing free and low-cost care to kids in need. But Mike didn't stop there. Over the ensuing years, he helped establish a new children's hospital, including a residency training program, and recruited faculty to teach new doctors the importance of public service in health care. His ongoing work included the development of programs for children with special health-care needs.

In recognition of his yeoman-like efforts on behalf of the neediest and sickest children, Mike was given a Distinguished Alumni Award from his college, an Alumni Citation Award from his medical school, and a Lifetime Achievement Award from the children's hospital he helped to establish.

One courageous patient, saved by one iron lung machine and numerous heroic medical caregivers, led to a legacy of thousands of ongoing miracles. Mike's life story taught us, and reminds us to teach others, the nearly infinite potential of each life saved.

EDITOR'S NOTE: When I (Dr. Rotbart) told Dr. Kappy about this "Miracles" book project, he told me the incredible story of a young boy surviving GBS thanks to an iron lung machine and many dedicated caregivers. That young boy was Michael Kappy himself, the co-author of this essay, who went on to the distinguished career described herein. Dr. Kappy noted that his story wouldn't work for the book because the doctors providing care for him as a child were very unlikely to be available to write about it, now sixty years later. I asked Dr. Kappy if he would allow me to help tell his story, and if he would co-author it with me. I hope you'll agree, this was a story well worth sharing on behalf of Dr. Kappy's doctors, nurses, and therapists of so many years ago.

10

Difficult Decisions

Patients and their families are often faced with gut-wrenching medical decisions, for which the right choice is far from obvious.

The first essay in this chapter describes the life-altering decision an extraordinary patient and her family had to make, confronting the very essence of life, death, and the meaning of both.

The other essays describe decisions where the fate of life or limb hung in the balance, but where seemingly impossible odds left only one reasonable and obvious choice. At times, fate seems to guide us to that obvious decision and it miraculously turns out for the best. But other times, the path not chosen may lead to the most remarkable outcome.

Choosing to Celebrate

Lia Gore, MD

As a first-year fellow training in pediatric oncology (the specialty treating cancer patients), I first met this eleven-year-old girl when I was called to the operating room by the neurosurgeon. He told me he had just removed as much as he could of a large invasive spinal tumor and thought that we would probably want to do bone marrow aspirations while she was under anesthesia to spare her the pain of that additional procedure. The bone marrow is where blood is made and is the frequent site where some cancers spread. As oncologists, we are frequently called upon to do bone marrow aspirations, removing a small amount of marrow through a needle inserted into a large bone, to evaluate the extent of cancer spread. Although this child's spinal tumor had put significant pressure on her spinal cord, and we were not sure if she would be able to recover the ability to walk, we were nevertheless hopeful that the emergency decompression surgery by the neurosurgeon happened quickly enough before permanent nerve damage had set in.

We sent the specimens from the tumor to the pathology laboratory, which confirmed our worst fear—she had a highly invasive *osteosarcoma* of the spine, a very bad type of bone cancer. Once the diagnosis was known, the supervising physician and I sat with the family for quite some time, talking somberly about the dismal prognosis for this disease. Osteosarcoma of the spine is typically not curable unless it can be completely surgically removed, and because of the location of her particular tumor, complete removal was impossible at the time of this surgery. It would have essentially meant removing her spinal column and several ribs through the midsection of her body. The five-year survival rate in this type of situation is less than 10 percent.

Her family consented to participate in a national research trial for patients with this diagnosis, comparing the standard therapy approach to more aggressive chemotherapy including an experimental new drug. The national center coordinating the research study assigned patients randomly to one of the two treatment groups. We felt somewhat relieved that our patient was assigned to the more aggressive arm of the study, hoping it would give her a better chance, but it was brutal therapy at best. She was in the hospital for the majority of every month, either for chemotherapy or for the complications associated with it. As part of her therapy, she also underwent a very complex surgical procedure attempting to remove all bones with visible tumor. We also elected to include a novel radiation approach during surgery. This complete process required eight physicians representing six disciplines and almost fifteen hours on the operating table with extensive spinal reconstruction (rebuilding the spine and portions of the ribs using synthetic materials to replace bone that had to be removed along with the tumor). We have since teased her that her back resembles the Eiffel Tower, which, in fact, it does.

Throughout her months-long ordeal, never once did she complain. Never once did she ask, "Why me?" Never once did her family waver in their commitment to making her experience as positive as it could be for anyone around them. This resilient young girl tolerated things better than anyone could have anticipated. Her family showed up in good spirits and decorated her room for every occasion and with every hospital admission. They took it upon themselves to bolster the mood of other families and patients, as well as all of us caring for their daughter.

About two months after surgery, we were horrified when an MRI test (a type of imaging study that produces pictures of the inside of the body) showed a large mass at the site of her primary tumor that had been previously removed. Again, we had a very long and, this time, even sadder discussion with the family. We were fearful that her tumor had not responded to our best attempts and that this most probably represented progression of her disease despite being on the very aggressive therapy. If that was the case, her prognosis was very poor and her survival likely would be on the order of weeks to a few months. We offered a number of options, and the entire family listened carefully and asked for some time to consider the choices. They went home with the understanding that we would meet with them again after they had had some time to think about all that we had discussed. We then decided together that we would repeat the MRI scan in a few weeks to see how rapidly things were changing, unless she developed new or different symptoms in the interim.

When they returned to clinic a few weeks later, we were all greeted by a beaming, jubilant young lady who had just turned twelve and looked like she had never felt better. There was no sign of spinal cord nerve damage or difficulty walking. Since we had last seen her, the family had decided to really celebrate her life, helping her experience things she would likely never be able to do in the future. They staged a prom. And a high school graduation. They went to Las Vegas to celebrate her "twenty-first birthday." They helped her live her life well and beautifully. We were very surprised that the repeat MRI showed that nothing had changed over the past few weeks. The large mass was still there, but had not grown larger. We had been certain that given how quickly the new mass had developed after the extensive surgery, we were going to see widespread continued growth of the tumor. We decided together with the family to biopsy the mass to determine its nature and try to predict how rapidly it might grow.

One of the surgeons from her first major operation performed the biopsy, and the findings could not have been more stunning to her or to us. The only finding was that our patient had developed benign swelling and inflammation in reaction to one of the synthetic materials that had been used in reconstructing her spinal column. There was no evidence of recurrence of her tumor anywhere!

Our patient completed her chemotherapy uneventfully. She continued to be a shining example of how infectious a great attitude can be. People flocked to see her, to hear what she had to say, laugh at the jokes she told, admire the ever-changing balloons that decorated her room. She joked that being told she was likely going to die got her some great trips for which she sincerely thanked her mom and dad. They all laughed about being able to do it all over again when the *real* events happened: prom, high school graduation, her twenty-first birthday. Never bitter. Never angry. Simply gracious and grateful.

To this day, she remains tumor-free. But the miracle of her story is not limited to her cure against all odds. This past fall, she celebrated what she has come to call her "Glad to Be Alive Day"—her sixteenth such celebration. Sixteen years from the day we told her she would likely die, and sixteen years since she chose to celebrate instead of succumb. Her decision to celebrate life came long before we knew she was cured. She was, and still is, at the center of an enormous ring of concentric circles of joy and sunshine that emanate from her wherever she goes. I've been blessed to watch her grow up happy and healthy, to see her graduate from high school, and then from college with honors. Every time I am with her, I am acutely aware that we all have choices in how we live our lives. More times than I can count, she chose to persevere where others would have given up. I and countless others have been blessed in so many ways by her presence in our lives.

I was a young trainee in oncology when I first met her, and she continues to inspire me to help others faced with similar choices of how to live their lives in the face of a dire diagnosis.

A Source of Light and Love

Daniel Hyman, MD, MMM

I met Melody and her family late on a Friday afternoon in March. I had just returned to work a few days earlier after watching my mom die peacefully in her sleep from ovarian cancer. I knew the experience of being with my mother when she died would change me and my perspective on many things, but I could not have anticipated it would happen so soon, or in this particular way.

Melody was born with *Trisomy 18* (T18), a genetic disorder that results in more than half of babies dying at or before birth, and fewer than 10 percent surviving to one year of age. Those dire statistics have understandably led us in the medical community to believe children with T18 will not survive and, therefore, to communicate with families of those children in stereotypical rather than individualized ways. But Melody taught me she was not a statistic.

When I first met her, Melody was thirteen months old and being admitted to our hospital for severe respiratory distress due to a viral infection. In the emergency department, the physicians and staff had discussed the situation and the likely progression of Melody's condition with her family. Based on these discussions, the family's understanding was that Melody was dying, and I was asked, and agreed, to admit her to my inpatient pediatrics service for supportive end-of-life comfort care.

As I walked into the room to meet her family and obtain a *Do Not Attempt Resuscitation* (DNR) order, whatever preconceived notions I had about Melody or how her care would proceed proved to be entirely wrong. That afternoon, with her loving siblings and their pastor in the room, Melody's mom and dad told me about their youngest child. Rather than painting a sad and pessimistic picture, they shared with me how Melody lit up the room when she smiled, how she interacted with those around her, and how her meal time was a special opportunity for her family to show her their love. Since her birth, Melody had become a central source of light and love for all of them, amazing them daily with some new skill or response. Her family considered her birth and her very existence to be a miraculous gift to them all.

Sitting in the room with them as Melody's family shared their feelings, I could not help but contrast those moments with ones I had experienced so recently when my mother's death became inevitable and imminent. My readiness to accept the death of my loved one, as painful as it was for me, was rooted in my knowing there was nothing more that could or should have been done for her. In contrast, if we simply provided end-of-life comfort care to Melody, I worried that this family would always wonder if they had done enough. Would they be able to find the peace of mind I had found?

I reframed the conversation with Melody's parents, asking if they were ready to lose her. They acknowledged they were not. They again told me Melody was a happy baby and brought joy to their lives; they truly wanted to be able to take her home again and were absolutely ready and willing to provide her with interventions that might help her to recover. I explained there were a range of treatments that might provide the support Melody needed to fight off her viral infection, yet were much less "heroic" than putting a breathing tube in her windpipe or hooking her up to a breathing machine. Knowing that with additional modest treatments Melody had the chance of surviving this illness and being able to go home again, they agreed to have Melody admitted to the pediatric intensive care unit (PICU) for supplemental breathing support. Admitting a child with T18 to the PICU inevitably raised some eyebrows among my colleagues, but I now felt I knew the family well enough to understand their needs.

I could not know for certain whether a period of giving oxygen under pressure through a mask, a non-invasive and painless intervention, would help Melody turn the corner, or whether her family would soon need to confront the question of further accelerating her support—perhaps to include a breathing tube and breathing machine—which would raise even more difficult issues. Either way, though, I knew that by trying to provide some respiratory and fluid support to Melody, this family would never have to question whether they had done all they could for their child.

Against all odds, simply receiving oxygen through a mask, Melody did beautifully. She never needed more aggressive care. She improved dramatically in the PICU over several days and then transitioned to home after about a week. I remember crossing paths with Melody's older sister on the following Sunday morning, just two days after Melody was admitted. The family had just returned from church and I shared my happiness that Melody was doing so well. Her sister said, "Well, there are many people praying for her, praise the Lord." Indeed.

Remarkably, Melody is now two-and-a-half years old, one of the rare babies with T18 who has lived beyond a year. And she has done much more than just live. She continues to bring joy to her family and community, a source of light and love. Melody's family has described to me how she has taught them all the concept of *agape* love, the highest form of love in which one gives to others with no expectation of return. Yet, without expectations, they have in fact received immeasurable return.

To her family, Melody has always been a miracle, and she has become one for me as well. I will never forget what she taught me both professionally and personally. Professionally, Melody taught me that in the setting of potential end-of-life decisions, which are never simple, understanding the values and perspectives of patients and their families, and discussing them purposefully, can guide our care. Her family has also helped me recognize that we in the medical profession have many preconceived notions about T18 and conditions like it, which can mislead us and cause us to communicate insensitively to families and incompletely with colleagues. Stereotypical language such as "incompatible with life" and "terminal genetic disorder" may keep us from considering even modest interventions we would not hesitate to offer to other children. We must always seek to provide patient- and family-centered care, and to do so we must consider every situation in the context of the circumstances and needs of each patient and family, rather than react reflexively based on a diagnostic label.

On a personal level, Melody and her family reinforced for me that there are times to intervene and times to let go, and they reassured me that I am still able to see the line between them and help others find that line as well.

I will always be grateful to this little girl and to this family. My wish for them is that Melody will continue to be their miracle for many years to come.

EDITOR'S NOTE: During the final editing and preparation for the publication of this book, I was overjoyed to receive a note from Melody's family announcing their celebration of her third birthday. In the text accompanying the announcement, Melody's family wrote this (reprinted here with their permission):

Everything Melody does is above and beyond what she should be doing. Melody's physical strength increases weekly, her coordination keeps advancing, her determination is remarkable, and her intellectual capacity is beyond anything we ever would have expected . . . Little Miss Melody, defying all the expectations, is still with us marching strong and blessing just about everyone she meets. She is a treasure, a gift, and a blessing beyond measure. We are so proud of Little Miss Melody!

The family has developed a website for all those who would like to follow her story:

www.MelodysStory.com

For more about Trisomy 18 and the risks of labeling, see:

http://www.brandonsmt18journey.com/
http://labeledthemovie.com/?page_id=14

An Impossible Pregnancy

Debra Gussman, MD

It was a beautiful Friday summer afternoon and I was anxious to finish work and get outside to enjoy the gorgeous weather. But as I got a call from the emergency room (ER), my heart sank. Friday afternoon phone calls from the ER almost always involve something bad for the woman they are calling about—and bad for the gynecologist they are calling. My first thought was, *Oh my . . . I hope this isn't a Friday afternoon ectopic pregnancy.* An ectopic pregnancy is a pregnancy that occurs outside of the uterus (womb), usually in one of the fallopian tubes (the tubes connecting the ovaries to the uterus). Ectopic pregnancies are medical emergencies that can threaten the life of the mother if not treated properly. It just seems like those happen more on Fridays.

I went to the ER and met Amanda, a lovely young woman in her early twenties. She was thrilled to be pregnant, but was having some bleeding and right-sided pain. After examining her, we did an ultrasound test (using sound waves to examine her abdomen) and, indeed, it was an ectopic pregnancy. I immediately took Amanda to the operating room to do a *laparoscopy* (inserting a flexible periscope-like device into her abdomen to get a close look at her anatomy) and discovered that the ectopic pregnancy had already "exploded," rupturing and destroying the right-side fallopian tube. Women have two fallopian tubes, one on each side, each connected to an ovary. Both tubes lead to the uterus. In a normal pregnancy, the fallopian tubes allow a woman's eggs to travel from the ovaries to the uterus where the eggs become fertilized by a man's sperm. In an ectopic or *tubal* pregnancy, the sperm go past the uterus, up into the fallopian tube, and fertilize an egg right in the tube. There is no room for a pregnancy to grow in the tube and there is no way to move a pregnancy that is in a tube to the uterus where it belongs. All a doctor can do when the tube is as damaged as Amanda's right fallopian tube was, is remove the bleeding tube, saving the mother and allowing her to heal, which is what I did. When Amanda awoke from anesthesia, she cried because this baby was lost. Her other fallopian tube, on the left side, looked fine and I thought she would still be able to have all the babies she wanted to have. After surgery, she healed well and was discharged home.

About a year later, Amanda came to see me again. She was thrilled to be pregnant. I examined her. Everything seemed off to a good start, but when we looked with ultrasound to see how far along in the pregnancy she was, there was no baby in the uterus. I took her to the operating room and discovered another ectopic pregnancy in her remaining fallopian tube, the one on the left side. This tube had not yet ruptured. I made an incision in the tube and cleaned the ectopic pregnancy out, hoping the tube would heal and she might have a successful pregnancy in the future. I was sad for her, but glad I did not have to take the whole tube out this time. That gave us hope she might still conceive.

Another year later, Amanda returned with yet one more ectopic pregnancy in the left fallopian tube. We were both so upset, but as difficult as this decision was, there wasn't anything else to do except remove her remaining tube to save her life. I was so sad to leave this young woman sterile with no functioning fallopian tubes. We talked in great detail about options, including adoption and in vitro fertilization. These were not good choices for her. She had limited resources, with no money for an adoption and certainly no money for in vitro fertilization, a very expensive procedure. After she was discharged, I occasionally thought of her with sadness, but didn't expect I would ever see her again.

Two years after that, Amanda appeared in my office, again pregnant! I asked myself, *How could this be?* I had personally removed both her fallopian tubes with confirmation from the pathology laboratory, where all surgical specimens are sent, that her tubes were, indeed, both entirely removed. We did an ultrasound, and to our astonishment and delight, the pregnancy was in the right place this time, in her uterus! I cannot imagine how her eggs could have made it to the uterus to be fertilized without fallopian tubes to get them there! Impossible? Yet it happened. Amanda considered this to be a miracle, and I couldn't disagree. She went on to have a very normal pregnancy and a normal labor and delivery. Her little girl was perfect in every way.

Amanda remained my patient for many years after that. She is a terrific mom, and she never got pregnant again.

DATE OF EVENT: EARLY 2000s

The Miracle of Good Information

Philip L. Glick, MD, MBA

Most referrals to my university-based pediatric surgical practice come from colleagues in the community or elsewhere at the university. This referral came from my rabbi, and the question he asked was not what one might expect from a rabbi. He needed my help finding an obstetrician-gynecologist who would perform a second-trimester abortion for one of his congregants. He told me that on ultrasound examination, this woman's fetus was found to have a *sacrococcygeal teratoma*—a potentially very serious tumor at the lower end of the spine. The woman's obstetrician told her that either the fetus or the newborn baby would very likely die, and recommended termination of the pregnancy.

I asked to see the mother. After much evaluation and counseling, and carefully reviewing all the risk factors, I advised the mother that I was cautiously optimistic. Considering all the findings on ultrasound and everything that had been published in the literature, I believed the advice she had received from her obstetrician was outdated and that the natural history for *this* fetus was favorable. The baby was *not* likely to die *in utero* (in the womb) or after birth, but would require major surgery very soon after birth. The baby would have a 20 percent chance of needing a drainage shunt to remove excess spinal fluid resulting from another birth defect frequently associated with the tumor. Shunts can have their own complications, including infection and obstruction, but generally are well-tolerated by babies and older kids. I also told the mother the baby would likely have problems with bowel and bladder function and may have difficulty walking because of impairment of the spinal nerves near the tumor.

After careful consideration, the mother and family decided to proceed with the pregnancy and hope for the best, recognizing now that this tumor was not likely to be a terminal diagnosis. The baby—a boy—was delivered by caesarean section with our pediatric surgery team in the room. Indeed, this very small baby had a very large tumor, equal to the size of the whole baby, on his lower back. Thankfully, my inclination was correct; the child lived, and the tumor was successfully removed surgically shortly after his birth.

As would be expected, he was left with a large scar from the procedure, and as he grew he developed a noticeable limp. However, he did not require a shunt to drain spinal fluid, and his bowel and bladder did not require major corrections. This was the best possible outcome, and we were all relieved this child had such a positive result.

This case proves that good information can make all the difference. Bad information can lead to wrong decisions and result in a devastating and tragic outcome. Knowing which information is accurate—especially in today's world, where we are bombarded with facts and figures—sometimes requires luck, or even a miracle, such as the highly unlikely path this mother took to the right information.

We don't always know what becomes of our patients but in this case, since the family's rabbi was also my rabbi, I saw this boy regularly at Sabbath services. Thus, I got to watch him grow, always greet me with a wonderful smile on his face, attend regular school, and become a vital member of a loving family.

I was fortunate to be in the synagogue for his bar mitzvah recently, on the occasion of his thirteenth birthday. I happily cried as he walked up to the pulpit to pronounce the blessings for officially becoming a "man" in our tradition. I have no doubt that, as an adult, this boy who very well might not have made it into the world will make meaningful contributions to his world.

DATE OF EVENT: 1981–1983

The Doctor-Patient Bond

Ann Schongalla, MD

Psychiatry residency training is different from all other specialties in that the relationship of the doctor and the patient is considered a fundamental treatment modality, along with medication, various psychotherapies, family therapy, etc. Great respect is paid to how to begin to work with a patient and, even more, how to end or "terminate" a treatment and say good-bye when necessary, for whatever reason. All residents (physicians-in-training) in all medical specialties have a built-in opportunity to go through this each year: on June 30 we finish a year of training and on July 1 we "graduate" to the next level. Of course, during a given year within our level we rotate on and off different services such as inpatient, outpatient, and intensive care units. Mostly, the good-byes are with staff we have become close with over weeks or months, because the patients come and go so quickly. In psychiatry the rhythm is a little different because the illnesses are chronic and have fluctuating courses, and what you're examining is how illness affects someone's life—not a body part or a lab test. The only way to learn about *bipolar disorder, schizophrenia, major depression,* or any serious psychiatric illness is to watch people go through it or, rather, accompany them through periods of illness and wellness during a long period of their life.

During my residency, our second year of training was spent working with hospitalized patients (inpatients) who were very acutely ill. We learned how to get their symptoms under control as quickly as possible so they could get back to their lives with as little loss as possible. Twelve months later, on July 1, we began our next year of training in the outpatient clinic where the goal was to learn how to keep patients with these same illnesses well and out of the hospital.

By and large, these were people with major psychiatric disability who were unable to work, and whose treatment was paid for by Medicare/Medicaid in our hospital teaching clinic. They were experienced in "getting" a new doctor every July 1, having to start all over telling their story, anxious about how well it would go with another new doctor. They were a colorful group with difficult, dramatic illnesses and we residents learned from hearing about each other's patients. At the end of that year, if we had time in our fourth and final year of training, we could continue working with a particular patient for the benefit of our education—often to the patient's great relief about not having to start over with another therapist.

At the start of my third year, in the outpatient clinic, one of my "new" patients was a man in his thirties with chronic paranoid schizophrenia who had a history of violence toward others, but was now symptom-free on medication. My job was to meet with him monthly if he was stable (or if not, as frequently as necessary to adjust his medications); to ask whether his medicines were working ("Hearing voices?" "Worried that anyone might harm you?" "Thoughts of harming anyone or yourself?"); ask about his medicine's side effects; and do everything possible to minimize his symptoms and help him live as unpsychotic a life as possible.

He was married to a professional woman, had two small children, and came from a college-educated family. Though also intelligent, he was prevented from getting a college degree or even a regular job due to his illness. You can imagine his feelings of humiliation. But you probably cannot imagine how frightening and *real* his convictions were of being followed and persecuted when he was ill.

Simply put, in schizophrenia, because of a mishap in wiring of brain tracts, people's five senses perceive what everyone else's senses do, but when they are ill, their senses also create false perceptions of reality. Only they experience that false reality and it powerfully overrides ordinary reality, especially if their senses "tell" them they are in danger. This is psychosis. You can't argue someone out of it. You try to protect them until their false perceptions and beliefs subside, and they are back with us again in the "real" world we all experience.

Forty years ago we had antipsychotic drugs that were reasonably effective but infamous for their bad side effects. So when I met my patient those many years ago, he was stable on medication, not psychotic, and we could chat about all kinds of things. But he was terribly sleepy and even dozed off in the middle of a conversation. He walked stiffly, his physical manner was eerily still, his voice monotone, speech poorly enunciated, and his face expressionless. Even if he said something humorous you could only hear it in the words. I prescribed all the usual medications to relieve these side effects—which caused their own side effects—but they remained disabling and humiliating. He knew the medicines kept his psychotic symptoms away, but he hated how the side effects exposed him anyway. He was damned with the disease and damned with the treatment—living not even close to a normal life. Nevertheless, he looked forward to his appointments, as I did, and he kept them regularly.

Imagine my puzzlement when, perhaps seven months later, he arrived for his appointment smiling, alert, physically comfortable with easy movement, talkative and engaging. When I asked what had changed, he said, "Nothing." He assured me he was taking his medication and had figured out how to manage the side effects. He denied any psychotic symptoms whatsoever. He came across as just a very ordinary, likable guy.

I said, "Okay, fine, if you say so. I am happy you are better but we still have to meet." He was happy to keep his monthly appointments, happy to feel well and to function much better. It was hard to say there must be something wrong with positive well-being. At the end of that year, he was happy to accept my offer to continue working with him during my fourth and final year of training. All continued well!

Inevitably and unavoidably, 365 days later, July 1 came around again. Having finished my training, I had to say good-bye and introduce him to his next resident doctor-in-training. We knew this phase of treatment would come and had talked about it, in a way, from day one. At our final appointment, he came in with a standard-size shopping bag filled many inches deep with full pill bottles—all the medicines that I had prescribed for well over a year when he looked completely well. But they had never been touched. No psychosis and no miserable side effects. He explained that he had filled all his prescriptions because he was afraid that the pharmacy would know and would call me if he didn't (okay, underlying paranoia). I was dumbfounded and speechless and, of course, worried because longstanding schizophrenia *doesn't* just go away and allow people to get off their medication. However, he'd been fine for so long off meds, clearly felt and functioned much better, and planned to keep up with his new psychiatrist, just as we had, to make sure he did not get sick. He had the right, and seemed moreover to have earned it, to continue to stay off medication. He was competent to make that difficult decision.

I really did not know what to think. What was he telling me with this bag of unneeded medication? Was it the way we worked together that stabilized him? Was it just a good phase in his disease? Had he been lying, and in fact had low-grade psychotic symptoms all along—most likely, I thought—that he'd been able to manage with his own cognitive behavioral strategies? What should his new doctor do to watch him? He said he did not tell me until the very end because he was afraid he could not be my patient in the medication clinic if he was not taking medication.

A month later I was filled with dismay and sorrow when I learned that his auditory hallucinations (hearing voices) and psychotic delusions of being persecuted had suddenly come back full force, including dangerous, threatening behavior toward others (which I had never seen or worried about with him). The police were called, and he was involuntarily committed to a long-term facility. Imagine what he and his family lost!

Now at the end of my career, I understand much more. I have seen many times how people with bad illnesses, even when taking their medications as prescribed, can fall apart in the face of great loss or change, even "good" change. Psychiatry is built on how talk therapy is fundamental to working through life stresses, with or without medication. Today, we also do much more *psycho education* where we talk about a patient's greatly heightened vulnerability to relapse when they are off meds and/or are faced with loss or change. We identify the *target symptoms* that signal relapse so they can restart medication—even a low dose—immediately (and then call the doctor). We may teach patients how to start a low dose anticipatorily when they see a life shock about to hit. With my patient who was stable on medication, today we might identify his early signals for relapse, and together—oh so carefully, given the history of violence—lower his medication to find the lowest effective dose that has side effects he could live with so that he would willingly take his meds. No way did he want to be a person who committed violence toward others. Simple things like getting regular sleep must be watched and safeguarded. Family members need to be the doctor's eyes outside the office. There needs to be more frequent appointments and check-in phone calls in between. And now we have enormously better medications, though not perfect.

There are many more strategies all with the goal of giving a person the knowledge and tools to control his or her illness. However, the basic illness of schizophrenia has not changed in its varying types, the particular symptom group of each type, the "positive" and "negative" symptoms, the variable severity and impact of symptoms on life course, and the wide range in responsiveness of symptoms to medication.

I am mindful that all treatment strategies work most powerfully when grounded in the healing effect of a relationship between a patient and physician, which provides comfort, companionship, and a safe kind of intimacy. That doctor-patient bond bears witness to life's difficulties and losses, and celebrates one's achievements and victories. It stands independent of curing. It is founded on respect and kindness for our patients and an abiding determination to help—even if nothing can be changed. And it gives as much to us as it does to our patients.

DATE OF EVENT: 2000

Ski's Legs

Bauer Sumpio, MD, PhD

Ludwig—known to his friends, of which I am proud to be one, as "Ski"—is a seventy-two-year-old man who retired to Connecticut in 2000. In his younger years, he studied at the RCA institute in Brooklyn, and during the Vietnam War he joined the Coast Guard, serving on their ice-breaker unit based in Alaska. After the war, he obtained a degree in agriculture from the University of Vermont. He was recruited by a giant computer technology company to work in their upstate New York headquarters, where he was an engineering manager for thirty years. His proudest claim to fame is that he was chairman of the committee of the Institute of Environmental Science that wrote Federal Standard 209, creating the guidelines for maintaining a "clean room" such as in the computer company's wafer manu-facturing plant, or in the operating rooms of hospitals.

I first met Ski in 2000. He apparently had been seen in a small hospital in upstate New York for complaints of leg pain, with his left leg worse than his right leg. The pain was present even at rest. Testing revealed that he had a large aneurysm of his abdominal aorta and severe blockages of the arteries in both legs. The aorta is the main blood vessel from the heart to the rest of the body. It runs from the chest all the way into the abdomen, where it branches into two major leg arteries, one for each leg. An aneurysm is a weakening of the wall of an artery, causing it to balloon out and, if not corrected, potentially burst. As Ski put it, "This was way out of the league of the doctors there and they recommended me to go to a large teaching hospital." Ski did his research and he chose to see me. I'm very glad he did because his story is one of my most moving and rewarding clinical experiences.

I am a vascular surgeon, specializing in problems like aortic aneurysms and artery blockages. At my first visit with Ski and his wife, I learned that his aorta was not the first blood vessel he had problems with. In 1995 he had a right-sided stroke that left him mildly debilitated. In 1996 he had a heart attack. That's when he finally stopped smoking.

Ski and his wife jokingly told me recently that they clearly remember that our first meeting together was in 2000 because "They were both non-Y2K compliant." In that one year, she was still caring for him after his stroke and heart attack, his leg pain heralded his severe aortic aneurysm and leg vascular problems, and she was diagnosed with uterine cancer! How much more "noncompliant" with good health can a couple be?

What followed was a long series of surgical interventions for a man who had extremely limited blood supply to his legs and, by all expectations, would likely become an amputee regardless of what we tried. I first repaired his large abdominal aneurysm by removing the diseased portion of the aorta and re-placing it with an artificial graft, a tube made of Dacron material. The graft, like the aorta itself, branches into two tubes, one for each leg. But the leg arteries were also diseased, the left side critically blocked and the right side on its way. I then did a *bypass* procedure on his left leg with another graft attached above and below the blockage, allowing blood to flow from his aorta to his entire leg despite the obstruction in his natural artery.

Unfortunately, this was not the end of his leg problems. Following surgery, he initially did well but then developed left leg swelling resulting from the reestablished blood flow into tissue that had been weakened or damaged from years of inadequate blood supply. The swelling caused what's called a *compartment syndrome* of his left calf, which threatened the survival of that leg—the pressure of the swelling inside the tight spaces of the calf can cause blood vessels to clot off and nerves to be damaged. We had to perform an emergent procedure to save the leg. We made two long incisions, one on the inner aspect of his calf and one on the outer aspect, to open up the four compartments in his calf that were under dangerously high pressure.

More trouble. Ski subsequently had serious infections with very difficult-to-treat bacteria underneath one of the incisions. The wound wouldn't heal and the germs burrowed down to infect the major bone in his lower leg. Infectious disease specialists recommended amputation for this non-healing wound with underlying bone infection. Ski, his wife, and I had long discussions of the best approach to take, the best decision to make. Understandably, he was very much against amputation, hoping instead for recovery after long-term antibiotics. But severe and resistant infections like this can spread from the leg to the rest of the body and be life-threatening. We all held our breath and decided together to stay the course for a while, observing him extremely closely and deferring amputation until it was clear there was no alternative. We would not let his leg infection kill him—but Ski made it clear that anything short of that was worth the risk of trying to save his leg.

I was out of town for a meeting when Ski developed a fever suggesting potential spread of the infection from the leg to the rest of the body. My covering surgical partner saw his leg and immediately began preparations for an above-the-knee amputation. Ski refused, saying he wanted to wait until I got back to decide. When I did return, we again together chose to continue his aggressive antibiotic treatment and wound care, including frequent surgical removal of dead or dying tissue. His fever and other signs of infection resolved, but we still weren't sure his leg was salvageable.

After eighteen days in the intensive care unit and fifty additional days in the hospital, he was ultimately fit enough to be sent home to the care of his wife. She diligently performed his wound care three times each day and I saw him as an outpatient every six to eight weeks. He remembers me telling him that the wound would have to heal "cell by cell." Indeed, there were times when it certainly seemed as if that wound would be there forever. Ski relied on his affiliation with the Veterans Administration to obtain his wound bandages and dressings, which he estimated would have otherwise cost him $100 per day.

After many, many months, the infected calf wound ultimately began to shrink in size and close, but there was a persistent drainage hole that seemed to refuse to heal, indicating deep infection might still be present. That concern precluded him from undergoing a left hip operation that he needed for yet another vascular problem in his hip joint that also threatened his ability to walk.

It took Ski's wound *six years* to heal completely. He ultimately underwent a successful left hip replacement and can walk freely, albeit with the slight aid of a cane. His blood vessels continue to challenge him. Several years ago I performed a right leg bypass procedure when the blood circulation to that leg reached critically low levels, again threatening the need for an amputation. Thankfully, this right leg surgery wasn't accompanied by any of the problems he had with the left side.

Ski now spends the summer with his wife in Groton, Connecticut, preoccupied with his lobster pots and fishing, his favorite avocations. He and his wife winter in Sarasota, Florida, and recently celebrated their fiftieth anniversary together. They enjoy the company of their two grandchildren, who are grateful for having mobile grandparents.

To this day, everyone who participated in his care marvel when they see him walking into clinic under his own power, some calling it "miraculous." After all, he's walking on legs which, by all accounts, shouldn't be there at all.

DATE OF EVENT: NOVEMBER, LATE 1990s

A Family's Prayers

Sandra L. Friedman, MD, MPH

Anna was a seventeen-year-old residing in a pediatric skilled-nursing facility because of extensive medical needs that made home care impossible for her mother. Anna had profound intellectual disability and cerebral palsy. She couldn't speak or walk, and she was dependent on others for all her activities of daily living. She required multiple medications and treatments for chronic breathing problems and a seizure disorder. She had to be fed through a tube in her stomach, and she slept with a special machine to help keep her lungs inflated.

Despite all these medical needs, Anna was an integral part of her nuclear and extended families and responded to familiar people with smiles and facial expressions. Her mother had emigrated from Southeast Asia and was very devoted to her care; Anna was her only child. When Anna contracted a lower respiratory tract infection and fever, she required antibiotics through her feeding tube. The first night of the infection, a nurse without extensive experience was doing the periodic checks overnight at the nursing home.

When Anna's blood pressure began to fall, the physician on call was not notified by the nurse and no additional care was provided. At the change of nursing shift in the morning, Anna was found in dire straits, with a dusky color, not responding to verbal or physical prompts. Her vital signs were severely abnormal with a weak and rapid pulse, and a barely detectable blood pressure. Paramedics were called to the nursing facility, and they transported her by ambulance to a local hospital where she required a breathing tube and breathing machine for stabilization. She was given fluids and blood-pressure stimulating medicines as initial resuscitation, but it was obvious she needed intensive care. She was again transferred, this time to a tertiary-care hospital.

Anna was admitted to the intensive care unit (ICU), where she was given intravenous antibiotics for presumed *septic shock* (blood poisoning), a condition in which multiple body organs are at risk due to widespread infection, as well as provided with continued support for her failing heart and lungs. An *EEG* (electroencephalogram, or brain wave test) was described as being "almost flat" with just barely detectable brain activity. The intensive care team recommended withdrawing support, as they believed her condition to be incompatible with life.

Anna's mother was confused and distraught. Uncertain as to the best course, she did not want to give up hope, and she reminded her caregivers that Anna had pulled out of serious illnesses in the past. Indeed, in the past, although others had questioned aggressive medical management for a young woman with such serious medical conditions then too, Anna had always recovered and returned to her baseline state of health. Her mother was concerned that withdrawal of support was being recommended too quickly in the ICU because of Anna's severe disabilities. Anna's mother felt that these doctors could not have known how important Anna was to her family, and she wanted the best medical care possible for her daughter. She was not ready to withdraw support.

Anna's mother called family members and close friends from the surrounding area and different parts of the country to come to her bedside. When they were all assembled, they prayed together at the hospital for Anna's recovery in a beautiful group service. I also found myself whispering under my breath, "Please don't let Anna die," as I knew how devastating it would be for her mother and family. With the support and encouragement of the gathered family and friends, Anna's mother decided not to withdraw support and her daughter continued to receive care in the ICU.

Slowly, as if in answer to her mother's predictions and prayers, Anna *did* recover. After a number of weeks in the hospital, she was able to return to the skilled nursing facility that had become her home; there she continued to recuperate. Remarkably—as if to remind us of how little we know as physicians sometimes—some months later Anna was actually functioning at a *higher* level than she had been prior to her illness.

Of all the health crises Anna had in the past, this one was by far the worst. Yet her outcome found her in better condition than before the latest illness began. Not only had none of the medical providers predicted she would survive, but we certainly couldn't have imagined her reaching a higher level of functioning than before. Anna would always have significant disabilities; however, she returned to the treasured place she held in her family just a little better than anyone could have dreamed.

Since that time, I have always wondered whether that prayer group turned things around for Anna during those dark days of septic shock. It certainly felt like a miracle to those doing the praying.

DATE OF EVENT: 1986–2012

Don't Feel Sorry for Samuel

Stephen Ludwig, MD

Sarah had died. She was a one-year-old with a rare metabolic bone disease that left her chest cavity malformed and prone to the failure of her ability to breathe. It was a tragic event for her mother and father, young parents filled with hopes and dreams for their baby daughter. They and little Sarah had fought a valiant fight but neither they, nor their doctors, nor the best that medical science had to offer, was able to help.

Shortly after Sarah's death, the parents called to say that they were expecting another child. They knew Sarah's disease was genetic but they were moving forward to build their family. I was happy for them but cautious, knowing that tragedy might strike a second time. The parents went for their prenatal checks and, despite their optimism, got the diagnosis they dreaded most. Examination of the fetal bone structure confirmed that the baby in the womb was also affected with the same rare and debilitating genetic disorder. Sarah's parents came to see me to discuss what we might do to try to avoid the same one- to two-year life expectancy predicted for this child, a boy. Had they considered an abortion? That was out of the question as it violated their religious beliefs, and their hope was that perhaps this infant would not be so profoundly affected. They would see the pregnancy through, and I agreed to do my best to support them.

Unfortunately, Samuel was born with the full, terrible manifestations of the metabolic bone disease. He had a dwarfed size and multiple bony abnormalities that gave his body a deformed appearance. Nonetheless, he had an alert face and bright eyes. Seeing him I could only think of the sister he would never know and wonder how a family could possibly live through the same trauma twice and still survive emotionally. I searched the literature, desperate to find someone in the world—a potential expert—who had treated this condition more successfully than we had for Sarah. One researcher from St. Louis had some ideas and we attempted a series of transfusions to restore the missing genetic material that caused Samuel's defects. The treatments failed. Due to his deformed chest wall, Samuel had more and more trouble breathing on his own. He was destined to die. Just like Sarah.

Meeting with the parents was painful and at the same time inspirational. They were such good folks and so willing to do anything to save their son. The question of a *tracheotomy* procedure (inserting a tube directly through the skin of the child's neck into his windpipe) and mechanical ventilation (breathing with the aid of a machine) came up in our discussions. They had seen this during the times they spent in the pediatric intensive care unit with Sarah. I had great misgivings, grave doubts. Ethically, was this the correct thing to do? Samuel would be tied to a breathing machine forever—however long that would be for him. Medically, was this the right thing to do? It was one of those decisions that you lose sleep over as a physician. What *was* the right thing to do for the child? For the parents? But as time passed, their resolve was strong. They wanted to move ahead and not risk Samuel's life; they felt they needed to do everything they reasonably could. They assured me they could handle it, and I agreed to support them in any way I could. I thought perhaps he would live for two or three years longer than his sister and they would have at least that much time together as a family.

The miracle unfolded over the years that followed. Samuel adapted to his *tracheostomy* (the tube now permanently in place in his neck) and his ventilator machine. Those bright eyes of a baby became the interactive smile and verbalizations of an infant and toddler. The family was incredible in their care of the child. His room at home looked like a mini intensive care unit. His parents knew how to manage many of the myriad nursing duties, and they had the additional help of skilled nurses visiting their home. The mother always knew where to find me in the case of questions or concerns. With all of this love and attention, Samuel rarely needed hospital admission.

As he matured, Samuel went to school with his electric wheelchair and his portable ventilator. He developed the ability to speak "around" his tracheostomy by managing an increased airflow to his lungs. As he attended his normal grade I began to see how right the parents were in their decision. He had intellect, wit, and a delightful personality. The kids in school graciously accepted him.

The family traveled with him, took him to sporting events, concerts, Disney World, and other fun places. As he got older, he was attracted to girls in his class and was a "groupie" for several of the female "rock stars," hanging out with the most popular girls, who enjoyed his company. He attended his senior prom and danced in his wheelchair. His life through high school was very normal despite a disease that was anything *but* normal. It was a very emotional moment for everyone when he graduated with his class.

Samuel lived to be twenty-five. He broke all longevity records for children with his disease. But more than long, his life was full in so many ways. Was it a miracle or just amazing care from his family? It was certainly a miracle in the eyes of his family—and a blessing; his parents did not have other children. His life touched so many others of us as well, for whom his life was also miraculous. For me, it was an honor to have been part of such a miracle.

Once, at a Phillies baseball game, his wheelchair was parked in the handicapped section next to a child who was profoundly developmentally delayed. Samuel said, "I feel sorry for him."

"Why?" I asked.

He replied, "Because he can't tell his mother that he loves her."

11

Silver Linings

Physicians are painfully aware of how often our best hopes for our patients and their families fail to materialize. Tragedy is, unfortunately, a fact of life in the practice of medicine. In the midst of some heartbreaking events, though, a redeeming and rejuvenating spirit emerges to help us through the sorrow.

For the essayists in this chapter, silver linings appeared in the darkest of clouds, giving them reason to carry on and helping them realize that not all miracles are physical or tangible.

DATE OF EVENT: 1989

The Miracle of a Single Question

Andrew Sirotnak, MD

As a first-year pediatrics resident (physician-in-training) at a large medical center on the East Coast, I was doing my final block of time in the neonatal intensive care unit (NICU). I'll always remember it was the week after the huge Loma Prieta earthquake in California—the one that happened during a live World Series broadcast and changed the landscape of so many people and places for the decade to follow. I had no way of knowing I was about to experience my own personal earthquake.

As residents in the NICU, it was our job to attend complicated or high-risk deliveries to provide initial care for the babies in the delivery room. I was called to attend a routine caesarean section being done because labor had not progressed. The mom was reportedly in fine health. The obstetrician asked for coverage from the nursery staff because the baby's heart rate had intermittently slowed down and there was concern that the baby might be born distressed. My supervising neonatologist (newborn specialist) was busy in a nearby delivery room with a set of twins who were quite ill, so I had to cover this delivery alone. This mom and dad were ready for the caesarean procedure and thought it would be like the one they had with their previous child.

As soon as the baby was born, the looks on the faces of the obstetrician and the delivery room nurse quickly told me this was not a routine delivery, and this baby boy was not normal. The baby was brought to the warmer bed for me and a nurse to resuscitate. I immediately recognized the tragedy that was unfolding there. Although I had never seen a baby like this, he looked just like the pictures in the textbook. The little boy was *hydrancephalic*, meaning his brain never developed and his skull was, for all intents and purposes, empty. His large head was almost totally translucent, as if it had been hollowed out. Hydrancephaly is one of the worst conditions a child can have, and it's impossible to survive from. It probably results from an interruption of blood flow to the fetus's developing brain during pregnancy. Without blood flow, the brain shrivels and disappears.

I knew this baby would die very soon. He already had severe breathing distress and was turning blue. The brain is very important in controlling almost all of a baby's bodily functions once out of the womb. The nurse and I made the very difficult decision to temporarily resuscitate the baby until the supervising neonatologist could arrive and we could have a discussion with the parents. The neonatologist was paged emergently to the delivery room. Mom was crying out, asking why she didn't hear her baby cry; Dad was asking to see his son. The nurse wisely asked the baby's father to wait for a minute as we helped the baby breathe. She then asked for another blanket besides the one we had the baby wrapped in, a request I couldn't understand until I saw her make a soft turban for the baby's head. The nurse and I looked at each other and knew what was next.

We called the baby's dad over and he knew something was very wrong. As he looked at his baby, I saw his fear melt into resignation. I had no idea what to say. *How do I explain this? What if I say the wrong thing? Why am I the one on call today?* But somehow, from somewhere, came this question as I took the father's hand and placed it over his son's hand and arms: "What is your son's name?"

He looked at me and quickly said, "Joshua, we think. Yes, Joshua. Like the story of Joshua and the battle of Jericho."

I had already known this was a very faith-based family, and the name they chose seemed very fitting. I then proceeded to tell him that Joshua was ill and would likely not live through the day. I explained that I would do everything I could to help them understand why, and I asked that we move Joshua to the NICU so we could make his short life easier. Late that afternoon, Joshua died. His dad found me as I was getting ready to leave the hospital and asked me to stay with them. I was honored to be able to stay with the parents in the mom's postpartum room, along with a large family who gathered to pray and comfort each other. They told me that my act of kindness—simply asking Dad his son's name rather than launching right into bad news or medical jargon—gave the baby's father strength to accept "what God had delivered to them," and the strength to support his wife. They kept the turban blanket and it was buried with him that week.

For me, my miracle was delivered to me that day by this family. I was a young doctor welcoming new life and then seeing the same life end in the span of less than a day. The family told me I had made some impact. This quiet, sacred, static moment came and went so beautifully. But it didn't end there.

Twenty years later, now as a supervising physician myself, I admitted a six-month-old baby from the emergency room with malnutrition, bruises, and overt neglect. His young parents had myriad issues, not the least of which were substance addiction, mental illness, and living on the street as transients. In the hospital, the baby recovered from his injuries, gained weight, and was going to be discharged to a foster home. On a Thursday morning before discharge, we invited the new foster family to join us for rounds with the baby's caseworker to hear the discharge planning. They told us how they had lost pregnancies, failed to be able to arrange previous adoptions through social services, and had finally given up hope of being parents. I quickly took the pediatric intern, my trainee, aside and suggested what she should say to this family, including what one question to ask. I explained to the intern that this foster family was taking on a traumatized child with an unknown outcome potential, yet they were looking to us for hope. We were privileged as care-givers to witness the formation of a new family—just as we in the delivery room do with a new baby. With the rough start this child had, he might have significant issues and may not turn out well. Of course, I knew that sometimes new babies in the delivery room aren't so perfect either.

We gathered as a team with the foster parents over this little boy's crib and started rounds. The intern began the discussion somewhat hesitantly, because the first question I had suggested she ask wasn't by any means routine.

She said, "We want to be the first to say congratulations on your new family member. We're here to help you understand what his needs are now as you take him home. Most importantly, what do you think his name might be as you become his parents?"

The baby's future mom started to cry—as did I—and then she launched right in with questions about his needs and care after discharge. I later bought a baby book and a card signed by the team as a gift, and mailed it to the family. Later in the month, that intern told me this was one of the most meaningful experiences she had to date in her career as a young doctor. I challenged her to carry that forward, as I had from Joshua. I told her our humanity as physicians must be embedded in everything we do for our patients and their families.

The new family successfully adopted the baby, and a year later adopted another son. Today, both children are thriving and happy. A letter of gratitude from the baby's new grandmother is laminated in my office. It comes in handy when I am not at my best.

Miracles are events that shock us with powerful awareness of something or someone other than ourselves, or other than the moment we are in at the time. That quiet, sacred, static moment that shocked me more than two decades ago as a trainee has never left me. To this day I call upon it and I try to pass it on.

DATE OF EVENT: 2003

The Miracle of Purpose

Dale S. Adler, MD

I came home late. My wife, Nancy, kept me company for dinner, as always. Our kids were doing their homework. As we cleared the dishes, I spotted a bar mitzvah invitation on the kitchen counter. A set of twins. I did not recognize the names. Nancy caught my quizzical look at the invitation and said she also didn't know the people or the kids, and she felt badly because someone was probably expecting an invitation and didn't receive it. However, Nancy was puzzled by the fact that the invitation was clearly to us, at our address. She feared phoning the senders, only to be embarrassed if, in fact, we knew the family of the twins. I stared at the invitation, and I thought for a few moments. Then I said, "I think I know who this is."

I met Harriet when she accompanied her husband, Ernie, to a clinic visit in the early 1990s. She was in her mid-sixties and Ernie was in his very early seventies. He had a strong family history of heart disease, was a former smoker, had elevated cholesterol, type 2 diabetes, and an extra fifteen pounds resting comfortably in his abdomen. Harriet recalled that her father-in-law, who had a heart attack in his fifties, made Ernie look absolutely trim.

About five years prior to this clinic visit, Ernie had a heart attack without warning involving the front wall of his heart. A *cardiac catheterization* test (injecting dye into the heart vessels to look for the cause of the heart attack) detected a blockage in the midportion of the artery that supplied the front wall of his heart. Unbeknownst to either Ernie or his physicians, and unapparent even on his EKG (electrocardiogram), the catheterization study also showed he already had a previous blockage of the midportion of the artery on the *back* of the heart. Ernie was staying alive on only one good heart artery, the large, dominant artery on the right side of his heart. He was taking effective medicines for his cholesterol and diabetes. Harriet said that her husband's arterial blockages could be traced to his mother, who filled young Ernie with fatty brisket, chopped liver, and magnificent cream-cheese pastries, and imbued him with the idea that hunger should be avoided at all costs.

Ernie loved to bowl, as did Harriet. They were a couple still very much in love. They had two married daughters, the older with a set of teenage twins; the younger, who married in her thirties, had no children thus far, much to the consternation and stress of both Harriet and Ernie.

Ernie had no heart-related complaints in the clinic that day, but because of the potentially precarious blood supply to his heart, he underwent an exercise imaging test that showed what seemed to be a stable picture. Sadly, less than one year later, he died at the bowling alley. He had thought he was dealing with the flu for a few days, and he wondered if he had a subtle gastrointestinal issue. At bowling, he simply said he did not feel well, became profoundly sweaty, and collapsed. The emergency responders came quickly, but resuscitation attempts failed.

Harriet came to the office as a patient herself soon thereafter. She was experiencing shortness of breath with physical exertion. She was still grief-stricken after Ernie's death. I learned that approximately eight years previously, she had received an artificial aortic heart valve for severe aortic valve disease. The aortic valve controls the flow of blood from the main pumping chamber of the heart to the rest of the body; hers was found to be *stenotic*, or stuck. She was in the 1 to 2 percent of the population born with a two-leaflet, rather than a normal three-leaflet, aortic valve, and she was in the one-third of those patients who had trouble with her abnormal valve. By the time she was in her fifties, she was having chest pain and shortness of breath when she simply walked across a room. Because of her ineffective aortic valve, her heart muscle was forced to overwork, and it hypertrophied, or thickened, like any muscle would if asked to do extra work. The thickened muscle demanded more oxygen than could be delivered by the blood vessels in her heart. Her heart developed scars in regions where there was a mismatch between blood supply and muscle demand. Her heart muscle was not receiving enough oxygen.

Harriet had a generally good result from the replacement of her heart valve eight years earlier. Her breathing improved and her chest discomfort disappeared. She was not perfect, however, for the heart muscle thickness only very slowly regressed. She was also not perfect because she was forty to fifty pounds overweight, had very significant high blood pressure and, like her husband, diabetes and elevated cholesterol. The weight, diabetes, and blood pressure all contributed to the thickness of the heart muscle and to the stiff blood vessels in her heart. They all also slowed any improvement of the thick muscle mass of the main pumping chamber of her heart. Though Harriet did not like to admit it, she actually ate as though she were being encouraged by Ernie's mother.

At that first office visit for Harriet as my patient, my examination of her provided rapid insight into this recurrence of shortness of breath, now eight years after the artificial valve had seemingly fixed that problem. There was an important leak surrounding her artificial valve. She had no signs of an obvious infection in her bloodstream that could be destabilizing the valve. She seemed to have the misfortune of what's called *late, insidious valve loosening*. Put simply, she needed another open heart surgery.

I should have known then that Harriet was no ordinary patient. At a lengthy re-operation, made difficult by severe chest scarring from the previous surgery, she was found to have an aged, infected, old suture (stitch). The infection was caused by a germ that usually doesn't cause problems, but in Harriet had slowly, over several years, gnawed away at the tissue that supported her artificial valve and kept it securely in place. The fact that she had done well for years, with an ongoing subtle infection, was actually quite remarkable.

After Harriet received her second aortic valve and a long course of antibiotics, her breathing improved again. But she was still not perfect. Nor was she even as good as she had been twelve months before the second valve. Her heart muscle was still thick and rigid due to the same factors as before. But now, in addition, she was experiencing complications of the second operation causing decreased suppleness of her heart muscle, the last thing that an already thickened, already rigid heart needed.

At age sixty-eight, Harriet lived independently, walked at a deliberate pace to avoid shortness of breath, and had already been admitted to the hospital a few times for heart failure related to her diseased heart muscle. Worse, due to her diabetes and high blood pressure, her kidneys were no longer fully efficient at clearing her of excessive salt and water overload. She had what we now term *heart failure with a preserved ejection fraction*, and she lived in a tenuous balance with her heart disease and her kidney failure harming each other in a vicious cycle. Her three- to five-year prognosis was bad—there was a much greater than 50 percent chance she would not survive five years.

After one of her several hospital stays, Harriet came to the office for a visit, and she had not a hint of discouragement over the need for her recent hospitalization. Nor did she lament her recent stay at a rehabilitation facility, where the food was never to her liking. Harriet was beaming. She told me that her younger daughter, the one who was previously childless and now in her late thirties, was expecting twins. "How wonderful!" I said.

Harriet filled me in on more details, saying, " . . . a boy and a girl, and the boy will be named for Ernie." I told her that I was thrilled for her, that she would have something wonderful to look forward to, and that she would really need to take good care of herself so that she would be able to enjoy the birth of these grandchildren. Harriet told me that I, her cardiologist, needed to take good care of her. I said that of course I would try. She said she didn't mean take care of her just over the next few months until the twins were born. She said that I had to take care of her so that she could be at their bar mitzvahs.

Inside, all my pleasure at seeing Harriet so uplifted quickly evaporated. The likelihood that Harriet could survive even to the twins' consecration, a ceremony marking the beginning of their Jewish education on their fifth birthday, was low. To survive to the twins' thirteenth birthday? With the severe heart and kidney impairments she had? Almost unimaginable.

The twins were born healthy and they gave Harriet a wonderful grounding. She told me how the boy named for Ernie was quiet, but a thinker, and bright. The little girl was also bright, but more mischievous. Harriet was exhausted on days that she babysat the children, who slowly grew into toddlers and were then even more exhausting.

Unfortunately, as feared, Harriet's medical condition was unrelenting. She had more frequent hospitalizations. She was part of the earliest hospital efforts to prevent readmissions by having home health visits several times weekly, and she even participated in an early version of telemonitoring. Harriet's medical condition was so dramatic, and instructive to doctors and doctors-in-training, it was presented at a hospital-wide conference as an example of the high cost of heart and kidney failure. The costs were not just financial—her illness took a tremendous physical and emotional toll. Her office visits became less frequent, but hospital admissions, including admissions to the intensive care unit, with the need for temporary placement on a breathing machine, became more frequent. Harriet was asked, as we do for all patients as severely ill as she, if she would want to be resuscitated if her heart stopped. She always answered, "Of course, I have to be at my twins' bar mitzvahs."

The years crept along. Harriet had to initiate dialysis for her failed kidneys, but she did so without complaint. She weathered a series of scalp operations for skin cell cancer. She lived through a severe *hemorrhage* (bleeding episode) that occurred when she critically needed dental work. She did not talk about her illness. She spoke about her twins. She was so proud of them. They were excelling in school. They were actually about to start their one-year-long bar mitzvah preparation lessons.

I think back upon the night I spotted the bar mitzvah invitation. Yes, one of the twins' names began with an E. I knew exactly who these people were. I told my wife the story of Ernie and his tragic demise, and of Harriet, who had looked forward to these bar mitzvahs, through extraordinary health vicissitudes, for more than twelve years. These were the bar mitzvahs that gave her life and gave her purpose.

We joyfully attended the twins' joint bar mitzvah ceremony, and it was a spectacular event. Harriet looked radiant, though frail. She was in a wheelchair, and she was now twenty pounds underweight. She had a beautiful wig and a wonderful pink dress. With the aid of a walker and an attendant, she stood and spoke to the gathered guests. She professed her love for her entire family. She remembered Ernie. She remembered the birth of the twins, and she remembered her vow—repeated many times—to see her twins have their bar mitzvahs. The twins talked about what they learned from a willful, loving grandmother.

Three weeks after the bar mitzvahs, her purpose fulfilled, Harriet died quietly at her assisted living facility.

DATE OF EVENT: 2006

The Thin Line Between Miracle and Tragedy

Robert J. Buys, MD

The dawn brought the beginning of the day we had worked so hard for, the culmination of a long and arduous journey to achieve a goal we once felt was out of reach. It was September 2006 on the island Kingdom of Tonga, located deep in the South Pacific. We were at last set to perform a series of operations known as *pars plana vitrectomy*, a procedure in which the fluid in the back of the eye is removed and the retina is repaired to restore eyesight. It was the first such mission ever attempted in this part of the world. We had a team of four: two of our best operating room nurses, an ultrasound expert, and me.

We arrived at the hospital with the bulk of our instruments not available to us. They were hopefully going to arrive shortly, after having been mistakenly diverted by the airline to Panama. We had salvaged some old instruments from the hospital and some basic ones that were sent to us from New Zealand to get us through the first two surgical cases. We had jerry-rigged an apparatus to allow us to use scuba equipment to run the pneumatic machine we needed to perform the operations. The money needed to make this apparatus had been donated for our trip by the grateful grandparents of the patient described in the "Shrapnel—I Knew He Had Lost His Eye" essay elsewhere in this book. All told, the value of the instruments we had to bring, via donations and any other means possible, totaled more than $400,000.

After our second case, my ultrasound expert told me that a patient we had seen earlier in the week in clinic for an eye examination had returned, having lost vision in his only eye. He was a farmer, a father of five, and years before had lost one eye from problems related to diabetes. He now was only able to see a hand moving in front of his face, a consequence of blood in the back of the eye that had just occurred in the two days since his previous visit to us. There was no view to the retina and hence the need for an ultrasound, which revealed a possible torn retina. I was left with a very difficult choice—we already had a full schedule and insufficient supplies to be able to add him to the list. We were forced to cancel a less urgent case and fit him in with hopes of saving his remaining eye.

It was miraculous that we were even able to help this patient. Of all the times he could have a torn retina, he gets it the only time a specialist team had ever been in the country, and at the exact time when we could operate on him and prevent a tragic outcome. The line between miracle and tragedy is a thin one.

But what made it really incredible is that I should never have been in Tonga on that trip in the first place. To understand why, I need to take you back in time.

Back to the day I died.

✧ ✧ ✧

When I was thirty-five, I noticed unusual beating of my heart and was subsequently told I had *cardiomyopathy* (a disease confined to the heart muscle and not related to any other medical problem). By age fifty, my heart rate was around thirty beats per minute (normal resting heart rate is sixty to eighty beats per minute), which I convinced myself was consistent with being in tremendous physical condition (which, given the extent of my exercising, was impossible, but denial works even for doctors). When my feet began to swell from excessive fluid I knew things had turned for the worse.

In the years that followed, my heart slowly, decisively, worsened. A pacemaker was inserted, and my exercise tolerance diminished steadily. In spite of this, or maybe because of this, I continued to lead my life as if nothing was wrong. Then came Athens and that fateful day.

It was a hot spring day and my wife and I had enjoyed the sights of the ancient capital. For dinner we went to the Plaka, an area around the Acropolis that was filled with narrow, twisting streets originally constructed to allow the Athenians to retreat and fight an urban war against an enemy unfamiliar with the layout. Now it is all about quaint cobblestone streets, a tourist destination. I went up to a gelato stand and ordered a lemon-blueberry.

I felt my heart beat very fast and irregularly. I bent over, and then heard everyone scream. Then everything went black. I would find out later that I had experienced an episode of *ventricular fibrillation*, a condition where the larger chambers of the heart beat irregularly and ineffectively. It is a fatal arrhythmia: brain damage can occur within minutes, death follows if it is not reversed. Somehow, my ventricular fibrillation stopped on its own. The line between miracle and tragedy is a thin one.

Well, that is the last time I ever order a lemon-blueberry gelato.

When I came to, there were strangers standing around me, I heard people saying my eyes stopped looking lifeless. That seemed like a good thing. I stood up, completely disoriented, confused. They called an ambulance which, like the Spartans of ancient times, was unable to find its way through the maze that is the Plaka.

The gelato stand owner was so happy to see me alive he gave me a free gelato just like my first order. If I had known that was going to happen I would have ordered a double the first time.

After that there were many episodes, too many close calls. I had a *defibrillator* permanently implanted in my heart that is designed to shock me out of dangerous rhythms like ventricular fibrillation. It's like having the paddles you see on TV, but inside you. It went off one time after I passed out while waiting for a green light to go on the freeway. If that had happened a few minutes later when I was on the freeway the results could easily have been fatal. The line between miracle and tragedy is a thin one.

One time I was in the hospital for observation while a new medication was being tried out to help my heart. I felt my heart race, my blood pressure fell to 80/40 (normal is 120/80), my lips and ears turned blue. I was barely holding on to consciousness when I heard "Emergency assessment team to room 7A stat" repeated several times. *Stat* means immediately, urgently. I thought to myself, *At least I am better off than that poor bugger.* Then it hit me: I *am in room 7A!*

They decided to take me to the intensive care unit. I called my folks; in my mind I was saying good-bye. I asked for a priest, I had to get something off my mind. When he arrived I was in *ventricular tachycardia,* another potentially fatal abnormal heart rhythm. I told him if I didn't make it out of the ICU he had to promise me he would tell my daughter, twenty-one years old at the time, to wear my wedding ring around her neck when she got married. Tell her I loved her with all my heart (and since my heart was massively enlarged to three times normal, that is a lot of love), that I was sorry I could not make it to her special day. That is what daddies do, give their daughters away, right? If I could not be there I would be watching. Right after that my ventricular tachycardia subsided.

In July 2008, only a couple months before the Tonga trip, my dad died. My hero and lifelong mentor was gone—he died from complications stemming from cardiomyopathy, the same problem I had. This shook me to my core and threw me again into multiple episodes of abnormal heart rhythms. Back to the hospital for emergency treatment with progressively more aggressive medications. By this time my Tonga team had done so much work; there were all the donations, all the expectations for the people of Tonga. I thought they were all lost, that the trip was over before it started. So did many of the people helping us. Then one of the nurses on my team came to me and said,

"I know things look bad, but let's just go ahead with what we have to do. Just another hurdle we have to overcome."

Inspired, I told my physician, "Patch me up, Doc. I have given these people my word. They are counting on me. Do whatever it takes to get me there."

In August of 2008, just three weeks before we were due to go, I experienced a shower of *floaters* in my eye, small particles in my field of vision. I knew right away I was bleeding and that the most likely cause was a tear in my retina. My own retinal tear; I swear doctors seem destined to get the problems they specialize in. I went to my ultrasound expert, the one who would travel with me to Tonga if we ever made the trip, and told him I had a miserable patient for him to examine. A real "dirt bag" of a patient, but try and be nice to him. Then I told him my name. He agreed with the dirt bag part, but saw me anyway.

Sure enough I had a tear in my retina, a large one. By some miracle it did not lift off my retina and cause a detachment. The line between miracle and tragedy is a thin one. I went to a colleague who had operated next to me for years; we both agreed surgery was required. I repeated for the second time, "Patch me up, Doc. I have given these people my word, they are counting on me."

Somehow everything hung together. My heart, my eye, my spirit, and off we went on our great mission, our great adventure. Thousands of miles away, to a land with rudimentary hospital facilities, where a vitrectomy procedure to save vision had never been done in their entire history. To a people we had never met, fulfilling our promise, against seemingly impossible odds we were going to meet our destiny.

✧ ✧ ✧

That brings us back to Tonga and the operation to save the only eye of the patient I described at the beginning of this saga. Ironically, he had a very similar problem to mine—blood in the back of the eye from traction on a blood vessel. We cleared out the hemorrhage, treated the problem, and by the next day he was 20/25, almost completely normal vision. To the best of my knowledge he remains full-sighted in that eye to this day.

We saw dozens of patients on that trip, helping to restore vision and, in the view of the islanders, create miracles they never dreamed possible. Such is the effect of what we see as our everyday practice of medicine in a part of the world devoid of such blessings.

After we returned home my heart continued to deteriorate, now even quicker than before. Soon I was told that I had no better than a 50 percent chance of surviving a year unless surgery was performed—a heart transplant, no less. I was stunned, speechless.

I was placed on a wait list; I had to wait until some young person died, in a manner that spared his heart, so I could live. And that really sucks. I should be the one to go and he should live on. When the call came I still could not believe what was about to happen.

Heart transplants are a big deal, with special surgical and anesthesia teams in place, lots of preparation on the part of the doctors, nurses, patient, and family. When that was all done, one of the doctors came in and informed us he was going to "harvest" the donor heart. He had a Learjet at his disposal and off he went at 11:30 that night. Then, all we could do was wait. My wife and I talked of superficial things, long pauses, and no mention of the surgery now only hours away. Finally, at 3:30 AM, the surgery team arrived and informed me it was time to go to the operating room. My mind quickly went to another hospital bed hundreds of miles away where the simple words, "It's time," meant saying good-bye to a fatally injured loved one forever as he was taken to the OR to donate his heart. To me. His trip to the OR meant death; mine meant life. The line between miracle and tragedy is a thin one.

I kissed my wife—good-bye?—and was rolled out of the room. I was alone with nothing but my thoughts. I thought of my kids, how lucky I was to have a loving wife and to be alive in a time and place where the miracle of organ transplantation is possible. How lucky I wasn't in Tonga, where even routine eye surgery was miraculous—what would the islanders think of replacing a diseased heart with a new one? We arrived in the OR and I looked around at all the instruments, the *bypass machine* that would allow the surgeon to remove my heart from my body but still maintain blood supply to my vital organs, and finally the surgeons, anesthesiologist, and OR techs assembled around the table. Ronald Reagan famously said when he went to the OR after being shot, "I hope you are all Republicans."

"We are today, Mr. President," was the reply.

Now that it was my time all I could think of was, *I hope none of you are ophthalmologists.* That was my last memory until I woke up.

I was back in my room. Everything looked the same as when I left. Did I really have surgery? Was it all some sort of weird dream? Then I saw the all the blinking lights from computer readouts, lots of tubes in my body, and to my amazement a cardiogram machine showing a normal heart rhythm. My first sustained normal heart rhythm in years. I turned and there was my friend, the nurse from the Tonga trip, who had never given up hope. My family had been up all night and had seen me as I came out of the operation, but I had no memory of it. I tried to talk, but could not; there was still a breathing tube down my throat.

And all at once it hit me, the operation was over. I reached out and grabbed her hand and in my mind screamed, *I'm alive!* I saw a tear roll down her cheek and she understood.

They pulled the tube from my throat, letting me breathe on my own, and I fell back asleep. The biggest day of my life was over.

The nurses told me that my first words after surgery were asking about who the donor was, over and over until they were sick of saying they could not tell me. Another memory lost to the anesthesia and pain medicines. The identity of my donor has haunted me ever since. But I do know it was a young life (someone said a twenty-three-year-old) taken far too early. My miracle was only possible because of the tragedy that befell my donor and his family. A thin line, indeed.

I feel I have not just another's organ; I have his spirit. I no longer refer to myself as "I" but as "we." I made a solemn oath that first day to take my donor, my internal and eternal brother, on the great ride that is life. That we would experience all that life has to offer together, for that is what we are. I would strive every day to be worthy of the great gift I was given.

For you see, there is a bond between us that can never be broken and a debt that can never be repaid.

We are one.

DATE OF EVENT: LATE 1980s

Redeemed

Bruce Reidenberg, MD

I t was the late 1980s in New York City and AIDS was a consuming concern. Young adults and a few babies were dying slow, painful, bleeding and choking deaths. I was a pediatrician training in infectious diseases at one of the few hospitals that offered a clinical research trial of the first AIDS antiviral medicine in children; it was called AZT (azidothymidine). At that time, the median survival for children born with AIDS was eighteen months. On my way to see a four-month-old boy with weight loss and worsening pneumonia, a very angry woman ran toward me and then turned down a hallway. She was cursing the nurses. She even tried to punch a nurse before she ran down the stairs and out of the hospital. A resident physician-in-training pulled me into a conference room and quietly told me that the woman was the mother of the boy I was about to see.

The resident said he called the infectious disease service because the resident was worried that this woman's baby had AIDS. I looked into his crib and the baby boy was able to smile at me. He was so weak and frail-appearing, we couldn't be sure whether he was developmentally delayed or just very sick. We did an extensive evaluation, adjusted his treatment, and confirmed that the baby had an immune deficiency, but we needed an HIV test to be sure it was AIDS. HIV is the virus that causes AIDS, and a positive test for the virus would confirm the diagnosis. For that we needed the mother's permission, but the contact information she gave the hospital was false.

Our wonderful social worker, with the help of local police, eventually located her. Unfortunately, she didn't come to any of the appointments or to the hospital to visit her son. After two weeks in the hospital, the baby's health deteriorated and he was transferred to the intensive care unit (ICU). The ICU brought him through a very severe pneumonia, requiring a very risky open lung biopsy, hourly adjustments of his ventilator (breathing machine), and frequent simultaneous dosing adjustments of several medicines.

It took several more weeks of hospital care for the baby to start gaining weight. Then the smiles became more frequent and he achieved some developmental milestones. His mother still hadn't visited and missed seeing him roll over for the first time. In the second month of hospitalization, she finally came to see him one night around 2 AM. The resident physician and the night nurse stated that she was intoxicated and belligerent. She wanted to take her baby home right then. She again cursed the staff when they suggested she stay at his bedside and learn how to give the medications and the special feedings her baby needed. The mother's cursing woke the other children and parents on the pediatrics floor, and there was enough chaos to require calling security. Around 3 AM, she tried to punch the night nurse and then ran out of the hospital. The next day our social worker was unable to find her.

The social worker had learned that the mother was a drug-addicted prostitute with no real address. Normally, the mother's behavior in the hospital would have brought on a formal investigation and the beginning of a placement into foster care. We were very concerned that she might return and take her son out of the hospital against medical advice and not care for him.

At that time, our legal option was to have the mother charged with neglect, which would result in her losing custody of her son. The hospital would then have the legal standing to use hospital security, and even police, to keep the boy in the hospital. If we did not pursue neglect charges, we would be partially liable for any harm coming to the boy through the mother's actions because we would have "failed to report" the danger.

The chief of infectious diseases shocked me when he argued for the mother to keep custody. At that time the only potential treatment for AIDS was AZT and it was not yet approved for use in children. The only way for a child to get AZT would be in our clinical trial that required parental consent. The chief knew that the government agencies would never give permission for a foster child to be enrolled in a clinical trial. The chief believed AZT was the boy's only hope for survival. I was strongly against allowing the mother to maintain custody and the right to take her son out of the hospital. I thought the mother was a more immediate threat to our patient's life than the HIV virus. If she took him home I was afraid she would not feed him, would not give him his medications, or might even give him heroin to stop him from crying. The chief overruled me and, with the social worker, made arrangements for the mother to have emergency housing and telephone service. Eventually the social worker and the police found her and moved her into the apartment. The social worker made an official "home visit" and declared it safe.

By now my patient was six months old and his mother had seen him only once since he was four months old. There was a flurry of activity to plan for the mother's training in all of the care that her baby boy needed. On the big day of the training and the discharge home, the social worker came to us to tell us that she couldn't advocate for the baby to be taken home. The social worker was upset because the mother had come to the office intoxicated and told the social worker she had sold the telephone for drugs. Without a telephone in the apartment, the mother would not be able to contact us if the baby's condition worsened.

The social worker told us that the mother was still in the social work office and did not want to come up to the pediatrics floor. The chief and the head research nurse rushed to the social work office to beg the mother to allow her son to be in the clinical trial of AZT. They were convinced that she understood it was voluntary and that the early results of AZT therapy were very good. They thought the mother was competent at that time to understand their cautions that AZT was not yet approved and there were unknown risks from the medicine. The chief was also certain the mother understood from that conversation that no child had yet survived AIDS. She signed the consent form with an X. Sometime later, she stepped out "for a cup of coffee"—and never came back.

For my patient, now on the clinical trial and receiving AZT, the next six months were full of deteriorations followed by small gains. Each time the chief and the social worker thought conditions were right for the baby to go home with his mother, his status worsened. His mother promised to visit at least once a month, but never showed. No other family members were known to our social worker and no one came to visit, even for his first birthday. We had a birthday party for him, decorated his room, and brought candy and some small toys. A few months later, we deemed him to be in his best state of health ever. Once again, the chief and the social worker made arrangements to bring in the child's mother, train her, have her take her toddler home and have a home assessment visit the following day. The social worker would confirm that the apartment was safe for a toddler and that our patient's health wasn't deteriorating. This time the mother showed up and was able to take her son home for the first time in almost a year. The follow-up visit was "acceptable," but three days later he was in the emergency room with pneumonia once again. Blood tests in the ER showed that he had not been receiving his medications. The chief continued to insist that we not report this hospitalization as "medical neglect." That way the mother could retain custody so that our patient could continue to receive AZT. If the mother lost custody, the government agency would probably rescind permission for the clinical trial and the

AZT would be discontinued. The chief argued that our patient was unlikely to be healthy enough for another trip home in the foreseeable future. Even if the mother had custody, the chief emphasized that our patient would be in the hospital, safe under our care.

Unfortunately, the chief's prediction about the little boy's health was correct and our patient deteriorated. He was transferred to the ICU where multiple simultaneous infections revealed that his immunodeficiency was progressing despite AZT. Today, we know that progression of HIV infection and AIDS almost always happens when only a single medicine is used, even when the medication is given as prescribed. Back then, AZT was not approved and it was the only experimental treatment for children. It became clear that the baby boy, now a "toddler" though he never walked, would die soon.

I was examining our patient in his crib when the social worker shocked me by saying that his mother wanted to have an appointment with me and the ICU doctor. The mother wanted us to meet her family. I had cared for my patient for more than half of his life and had never seen any family other than his mother. Surprisingly, the mother showed up on time and sober. She brought her sister and a fifteen-year-old she introduced as my patient's half-brother. The mother's sister was an angry-appearing woman in a wheelchair with a below-the-knee amputation of her right leg. The teenage half-brother was stony faced, wearing baggy clothing, and kept his right hand in his pocket. I was frightened of him because I thought he might have a gun in that pocket. We went to the little boy's crib so his aunt and half-brother could see him, possibly for the first time. The ICU doctor and I showed the family that our patient was unconscious and that his spontaneous movements showed he was in no pain. We described the function of all of the machines being used to maintain his comfort, and we talked about his declining health. Both the aunt and the half-brother appeared angry, so the mother said we should move to the family room away from the crib.

The next moments are fixed in my memory. The mother said to her family members, "I brought you here to tell you a few things. First, these doctors and nurses have worked so hard to care for my son. I know there's nothing they could do to prevent his death. Second, when he dies, I want him to have an autopsy. I don't want anyone to suffer the way my son has. I'm telling you this now because I don't know if I'll be around when he goes, so you need to know this is what I want."

At this point, the aunt yelled, "I don't want him to have no cut-up exam!"

The mother said, "He's going to have it. I will sign any forms. The docs need to know what happened to him so that other kids won't suffer." Then the mother looked at her teenage son who had not moved or made any sound. She asked, "Do you understand?" He nodded. Then there was a long silence as all three family members stared at the floor. Without any other word to us or to each other, they filed out and left the hospital. I found a quiet place alone and cried.

About a week later our patient died. His death was peaceful and he had no pain, but there was no family present. After we declared him dead, the social worker produced the mother's letter insisting on an autopsy. The autopsy was done promptly; the results were fascinating and instructive for us. About one month after our patient died, his mother insisted on an appointment so that she could understand the autopsy results. She arrived on time and sober. We thanked her for the kind things she said about us to her family. We described what we had learned from her son and how that would change how doctors will care for future patients. When she left the room she was crying, but with a Mona Lisa smile on her face.

One month later, the social worker gave me a handwritten thank-you note from the mother. It had her real signature, not an *X*. I later learned that she spent the following six months talking to school groups about HIV and AIDS. Then she died from her own AIDS. Her thank-you note is a treasure I've kept for decades as proof that this transformation, this redemption, really happened.

DATE OF EVENT: EARLY 1990s

The Tears We Shared

Clara Escuder, MD

She was a beautiful, petite baby, born into a very religious African-American family in the large East Coast city where I was in private practice. From the beginning we knew something was wrong—she held her fists too tightly clenched and had a very tiny mouth. We later learned Baby M had a genetic condition called *trisomy 18*, an extra chromosome in every one of her cells. I spoke with genetics experts at the university hospital and learned that Baby M's condition was grave and most babies with this defect do not survive to their first birthday. I had never had a patient with this condition and rapidly became very bonded to this wonderful and loving family.

Baby M had difficulty with feedings and gained weight very slowly. We discovered she had a heart condition, not uncommon in babies with trisomy 18. During those first days and weeks of her life, after a busy office day, I often spent time talking with her parents, discussing their concerns and fears. This was therapeutic for all of us—her parents were able to ask questions, cry, and express their deep love for their new baby. In turn, I was able to feel I was offering something to them when, in fact, there was so little I could do medically for their baby.

My time with Baby M was very brief. She died at three months of age. Her heart couldn't hold on any longer. The nurse I worked with and I attended the funeral service at a local church, which was filled to overflowing with friends and family. There was such an outpouring of support and love, it was electric. Baby M looked as peaceful and beautiful as the day she was born, showing no evidence of the disarray inside her little body. We were the only non-African-Americans there, relevant only as an explanation of why I was noticed. Well, it wasn't the only reason. I could not stop crying throughout the service. I sobbed and sobbed and sobbed. My heart was breaking for this family, and I felt I had not done enough for them or for their baby. I didn't realize at the time how noticeable my anguish had been.

Two years later I was notified by the university hospital that a family had requested I see their newborn baby boy in the nursery and asked that I become his pediatrician. As community pediatricians, it is not unusual to be called by the hospital to tell us of a new patient headed for our practice, but often that's either by a random assignment by the hospital based on neighborhood, or following interviews with the family prior to the baby's birth. It was unusual to be specifically requested by a family unfamiliar to me. I went to the hospital after office hours and met the new parents and baby boy—a handsome, robust little guy. I didn't recognize the family and was sure I had not met them before. But the baby's father said he had seen me before; he was the pastor at Baby M's service, and he was also Baby M's uncle.

After his niece's funeral two years earlier, Reverend E asked his brother, Baby M's father, who that woman was who could not stop crying. His brother answered, "That's our pediatrician."

The pastor told his brother, "The day I have a child, I want her to be our pediatrician."

During our training in medical school and residency, we often get the message, either directly or tacitly, that we have to be tough to get through the challenges and traumas of training and the practice of medicine. We need to separate ourselves from our emotions, never cry, "Be professional." I learned with this dear family that tears and compassion are not a sign of weakness, but a sign of tenderness and caring and being human. The tears we shared, this family and I, created a lifelong bond between us. When my mother passed away twenty years ago, Reverend E came to the funeral with all three of his children—my patients—dressed in their Sunday best.

I moved away from that city ten years ago, but Reverend E still calls me several times a year to say hello, to see how I'm doing, and to share the news of his now-grown children, Baby M's first cousins, whom I had the privilege of caring for.

EDITOR'S NOTE: For another touching perspective on trisomy 18, as well as references for additional information on that condition, see the essay titled, "A Source of Light and Love" elsewhere in this book.

DATE OF EVENT: 1980

A Child's View

Edward J. Goldson, MD

I n the practice of medicine, sometimes heartbreaking events take place. Adults, including caregivers and parents, often have trouble knowing how to respond to unexpected and potentially tragic circumstances. A lovely couple delivered their second, much-wanted and much-anticipated child: a full-term, good-sized, apparently healthy baby boy.

Although the baby had the right number of legs, arms, fingers, and toes, and was breathing normally with a good heartbeat, the shock came quickly when the doctors and nurses took a closer look. The left side of the baby's head was devastatingly deformed with a large *encephalocele* (a profound defect in the skull exposing part of the brain). The baby also had a large facial defect, a gaping opening extending from the mouth almost to the left ear.

The doctors and nurses were saddened, understanding the implications of this horrific birth defect—multiple restorative surgeries with the possibility of brain damage, developmental delays, and even death. Needless to say the parents were devastated! After dealing with the immediate shock, the next question was how were they going to tell their five-year-old daughter about her brother, and should she even be allowed to see him? She had been so excited to have a baby brother and couldn't wait to meet him! Much discussion ensued among the doctors, nurses, social worker, and parents. Ultimately, the family decided their little girl should be brought to the nursery and introduced to her baby brother.

With great trepidation on the part of all of us involved, the day arrived for the big sister, accompanied by her parents and the family physician, to visit the baby. The little girl didn't seem to be much bothered by the adults who acted as if they were walking on glass shards as everyone entered the nursery. She curiously approached the bassinet, took a very thorough look at her baby brother, and said, "He's cute!" There wasn't a dry eye in the room among the medical staff observing the simple yet wonderful response of this lovely child.

On that day, we were all reminded of the miraculous ability of children to teach adults how to be human and accepting.

DATE OF EVENT: 1997–PRESENT

The Miracle of Resilience

Simon J. Hambidge, MD, PhD

Some miracles are born out of tragedy. As a freshly minted supervising pediatrician at a large urban practice delivering care to low-income, uninsured, and vulnerable populations, I provided care to a newborn I will call Juan. He was a beautiful and healthy baby, his parents' first child. His parents were not well-off, but his father worked two or three jobs at a time to support his new family.

At the age of four months, Juan developed seizures and stopped reaching his developmental milestones. Although he was given a number of diagnoses, including *infantile spasms* (a severe type of seizure disorder) and *cerebral palsy* (or CP, a muscle and movement disorder), these were merely descriptive of his symptoms. We couldn't determine the underlying cause of his condition, despite many, many tests. Early on, when Juan had only had a couple of seizures associated with fevers, I offered reassurance to the family, but my reassurances turned out to be false.

By the age of six to seven months it was clear that he was not going to be the boy that his parents imagined and hoped for. Their pain was palpable. They wanted to know why this had happened to their son, and appropriately wanted everything done to figure out his diagnosis. One of my biggest challenges as a young pediatrician was dealing with the limits of medicine to provide the answers they were looking for. Throughout this time, they were never angry or resentful, and they kept their energy focused on what was best for Juan.

Over the next nine years, although Juan had profound developmental delays, could not communicate verbally, and was confined to a wheelchair, his mother provided incredible care to him, and he was able to interact with her in simple ways. It seemed possible to tell his emotions, and the family did everything they could to make him happy, including exploring unconventional therapies, such as swimming with dolphins and riding horses. I saw him numerous times every year, and all our clinic staff knew the family well. I was always struck by the deep relationships both parents had with Juan, and how he seemed to be such a happy child despite his profound disabilities.

As he grew older, his ability to handle his own secretions diminished, and he developed recurrent pneumonias from the accumulation of those secretions in his lungs. In his last year of life, when it became clear he would not survive much longer, I began to have conversations with his parents about alternatives at the end of life, and especially about the futility of heroic interventions (breathing tubes and breathing machines) when the lungs are so damaged that there is no possibility of recovery. Juan's mother (who by this time was essentially providing home intensive care for him) understood this and did not wish to intervene further. But his father had a much harder time letting go, and for a time wanted "everything done." One of my biggest learning experiences at that time was helping them navigate their different wishes. Both parents loved Juan deeply but were at very different points in their acceptance of his ultimate prognosis. By this time Juan required a breathing machine in the hospital. Eventually, his father decided that he "did not want to see Juan suffer anymore" and the parents requested to have all mechanical breathing equipment removed. He died peacefully at age nine with family, physicians, and nurses in attendance. I was there that afternoon as Juan was taken off of his ventilator. His breathing slowed, and slowed some more, and he was serene and tranquil in his parents' arms as he died. There were many tears—tears of sorrow, but also tears of happiness for a young boy who had been able to impact the lives of so many people, and to live to his maximum potential because of the love and devotion of his parents. Still, the loss of their beautiful boy and all the potential he embodied at birth was a tragedy for Juan's family.

Yet out of that tragedy emerged a miraculous resilience. I am still closely involved with Juan's family eight years later, providing care to his three younger sisters. The oldest of the three remembers him; the other two were born after his death. But Juan lives on in all their memories, kept alive by a houseful of pictures and their family storytelling. And they are happy memories. His family celebrates his brief life and does not dwell on the many challenges he and they faced, or on their ultimate devastating loss.

Juan's life and death had an especially powerful impact on the oldest of his three younger sisters, the one who can remember him. She now attends a tough inner-city high school, but does well and is focused on her dream of becoming a nurse or doctor; she wants to specialize in pediatrics. If her memory of Juan can inspire her to pursue her dreams and become a pediatrician, ultimately caring for young children like her brother, that will be yet another example of the miraculous resiliency of this family in the face of tragedy.

Being privileged to watch the family cope over all these years, it would be something of a personal miracle for me to see Juan's sister become a pediatrician. I have told her I will mentor her in any way I can.

DATE OF EVENT: JANUARY 2006

The Miracle of Forgiveness

Harvey Guttmann, MD

I t was going to be a routine procedure to help my patient swallow food with greater ease. We had known each other for a few years, but not particularly well. Hilda was in her late sixties and had struggled with severe asthma most of her life. I had seen her previously to dilate her esophagus (food pipe) when she was experiencing difficulty in swallowing. She would develop a narrowing of her esophagus every one to two years from stomach *acid reflux* (backflow of stomach juices up into the esophagus) and would come to me for a "stretching" procedure with a balloon-type dilator inserted into her esophagus through her mouth. I had performed this without any complications many, many times before, and at least three or four times on Hilda herself.

That day, however, what began routinely ended up horribly wrong. Within a minute or two after the stretching was completed, and even before fully awakening from her anesthesia, Hilda's breathing became labored and she clutched her chest in excruciating pain. It became quickly apparent that instead of uneventfully dilating the esophagus, the procedure had resulted in a serious tear. I watched in horror and disbelief as the emergency resuscitation "code team" of doctors and nurses was called over the hospital loudspeaker. They ran to our procedure room and placed both a tube through the chest wall and a breathing tube into the trachea (windpipe) of my patient, who a mere fifteen minutes earlier was joking with me prior to the procedure. She was quickly rushed to the operating suite and, because of the severity of the tear, the esophagus needed to be removed in its entirety.

The ensuing weeks were a blur to my patient, her family, and to me. Hilda required the breathing tube for nearly two weeks after surgery and the chest tube for a month. One complication led to the next. I awakened each morning thinking of my poor patient and went to sleep praying for her recovery. I visited her and her family twice daily in the intensive care unit but could not communicate with her because of the breathing tube in her windpipe and the sedation that was administered to maintain her calm.

When she was first able to speak to me, she was short of breath and uncomfortable but over the ensuing two-month hospitalization, her breathing slowly became less labored, allowing her the strength to talk. Although she inquired about the details of the complication, she never expressed anger toward me, and for that kindness, I was most thankful. As she continued to gain strength she would share her feelings during our daily visits, not only regarding her acute medical situation or her chronic breathing issues, but about her family struggles, her career, her life's victories and disappointments. Her eyes twinkled with joy as I entered the room, and we both began to look forward with anticipation to those daily chats as the highlights of our day.

My emotions were mixed and confused when the time arrived that she was well enough to leave the hospital. We had developed a relationship that soothed our souls. Each time we sat together in conversation, I could see her breathing becoming visibly more comfortable as the visit progressed. We shared the Jewish faith and, although neither of us was ritually religious, each Friday over the ensuing four years following that hospital stay, I would call her home in the afternoon to wish her a Sabbath greeting. When she answered the phone, I believed I could feel her smile through her shortness of breath, and by the end of each weekly chat, she was coughing less forcefully and her voice was much stronger—as was mine. We both began each Sabbath feeling spiritually and physically invigorated.

But the years of illness, along with the added stress of the procedure's tragic complication, took their toll on my patient's ability to breathe. With the passage of time, I stood witness each Friday to the dwindling force of her breaths as they gradually became more labored. The initial improvements I observed early on during our pre-Sabbath conversations became less apparent to me as the years passed, despite the fact that our connection to each other became increasingly close.

What began as a horrific and life-altering complication evolved into a miraculous and life-affirming bond of friendship. But, as her decline continued relentlessly, she required another admission to the hospital. It was then that she shared with me her feelings that the time had finally come for her to say good-bye. She could no longer fight so hard each and every day to fill her lungs with air, and it was time for her to transition to hospice care. With her family and me at her side, and with the help of her compassionate nurses, she slowly drifted toward unconsciousness and passed away comfortably, surrounded by those who loved her.

Who could have believed that despite this tragic complication, she would survive the years, and how fortunate for us all that she could. Did those Sabbath greetings help gather and maintain her strength to live? Although I cannot ever be certain, I want to feel as if they had. They certainly gave me strength and comfort. And so, during her last days with us, I was honored to be able to wish her one final Sabbath farewell.

To this day, each Friday as the Sabbath approaches, I close my eyes in reflection and offer my dear departed friend and patient another greeting for the miracle of forgiveness and gift of friendship that she gave me.

DATE OF EVENT: APRIL 2000

A Child's Insight

David Keller, MD

The "Father of Modern Medicine," Dr. William Osler, once said: "Listen to your patient. He is telling you the diagnosis." As a pediatrician, I tried mightily to adhere to that guidance as I attended to the nuances of the lives of my patients in the small New England town where I practiced. I listened to many stories from my families. Usually, I was able to glean from them the information I needed to make a diagnosis. Before I listened to Bob, however, I hadn't truly appreciated that pediatricians' patients are not limited to just the kids in the exam rooms, but include their families as well. We have to listen to all of them.

I first met Bob as he was entering elementary school. He had cerebral palsy, a movement and muscle problem that results from damage to a baby's developing brain. This young boy also had speech problems and significant learning disabilities which, along with his cerebral palsy, were the result of a rocky start in life as a thirty-two week premature infant. His condition was not severe enough to need crutches or a wheelchair, but was bad enough to keep him from running with the other kids. He wore plastic braces on his lower legs to prevent his muscles from permanently shortening due to their chronic spasms. When he walked, it was obvious his condition would make it difficult for him if he ever wanted to participate in an athletic activity. His speech was hard to understand, and he had few friends.

By second grade, it was clear that school was going to be a challenge. I spent many hours talking with his mother, working with her to get special-education services at school to supplement the physical therapy he was receiving to minimize the impact of his cerebral palsy. In fifth grade, we (his mother, the school, and I) decided that Attention Deficit Hyperactivity Disorder (ADHD) might explain some of the problems he was having in class. Kids with ADHD may have trouble paying attention, may act without thinking about what the result will be, and may be overly active. For reasons that aren't fully understood, medicines that *increase* activity in most people (stimulant medicines) will help *decrease* hyperactivity in kids with ADHD. We decided to start Bob on stimulant medicine to see if it would have a beneficial effect on his ADHD.

Throughout this time, I spoke with Bob as a child, thinking of his mother as the primary source of information about his progress. Even though I saw him and his mother frequently, I often "spoke past" him when addressing his condition with his mom. I still saw him as an awkward lad, with an odd affect, difficult speech, and a funny gait, who would always be a child dependent on his mother.

In high school, Bob encountered new challenges in the education system, struggling in all subjects and failing despite medications and school support. When he came in for his annual physical, for the first time he refused the stimulant medications that had been prescribed. In the room with his mother, I heard her speak of being at the end of her rope. From him I heard nothing. I asked his mother to step out of the room, so that I could examine this teenager in privacy.

"So, what's going on?" I said as I began my examination. He said nothing. I probed further, "The pills never bothered you before."

"They don't work," he replied, "and I don't want them around the house."

I stepped back from the table, surprised by his response. "Why not?"

"She's drinking again," he replied, "and I don't want her to start with the pills."

Suddenly, it clicked. In retrospect, his mother's *affect* (a psychological term, meaning one's outward presentation of inner emotions) was often a bit tipsy. I had written it off as stress. I knew that she had been divorced and suffered from depression. I didn't know that she had a problem with drinking or pills. It had not occurred to me that her fifteen-year-old, special-needs son would realize that restricting his mother's access to his stimulant medication was what he could do to keep her problem from getting worse. His insight gave me a chance to help him have a conversation with his mom that was long overdue. The ongoing dialogue they established helped them both in ways I could not have anticipated—certainly more than any change I could make in his prescription.

Bob's school performance improved. Now that we knew of his mom's drinking, we were able to help her get treatment, and her drinking came under control. Bob was able to stay on his medication without worry that his mom would be tempted. All this was the result of the unexpected and, in my eyes at least, somewhat miraculous perceptiveness of a child to whom I had not given enough credit.

Over the next few years, we decreased and finally eliminated Bob's stimulant medication. At each visit, Bob and I always had a private conversation as part of the visit. I now knew to speak with him as a young adult, not past him as a dependent child. I respected his self-awareness and wisdom. After each visit, I always made sure to ask his mother how she was doing in her work on recovery, and she always thanked me for asking.

Bob graduated from high school, an incredible testimony to his perseverance and maturity. Although he would still probably always need assistance in life, there was no doubt he was ready to transition to an adult world. I'm certain his intuition and understanding will surprise others as it had surprised me.

DATE OF EVENT: 2015

Feeling His Pain

Jeffrey S. Hyams, MD

I t was a routine follow-up office visit for Anthony, a fourteen-year-old boy I had seen for several years for *eosinophilic esophagitis*. This is a condition in which allergy to a food protein causes inflammation in the esophagus, the tube leading from the mouth to the stomach, causing difficulty swallowing. Anthony had been doing well on moderate dietary restriction when I last saw him six months previously. I asked him the customary questions about how he was doing, but could sense that I was not getting the whole story. As he was old enough to talk to me directly, without his mother participating in the conversation, I directed my questions to him.

Over the next few minutes it became clear that while his esophagus was fine, Anthony was not. He was having abdominal pain, diarrhea, fatigue, and not doing as well in school as usual. I did the customary head-to-toes "review of systems," methodically asking about any physical symptoms or other issues he was having. I then asked him more about his life, school, home, stresses, and the like, but really didn't get much in return. Mostly he stared at the floor. Finally I turned to his mother, herself a nurse, and asked if she had anything to add. Anthony's mom was the kind of person who was always smiling, but not today. She told me that her husband had been quite ill for many months with a yet-to-be-defined illness that had left him incapacitated. Their world had been badly shaken. He was being cared for at home but clearly the demands of his illness on her, and on Anthony, had been great. I was very fond of this family as we had shared stories of our lives on previous visits and I didn't want to offer platitudes. I wasn't sure exactly what was right to say at that moment, though I knew what I wanted to say.

What I wanted to say was that I had lived in their shoes for many years with my first wife being progressively disabled, and then eventually dying, from multiple sclerosis. What I wanted to say was that I, along with my teenage son, had been my wife's caretakers and we saw the incremental impact of her illness on us. My son and I had experienced anguish, stomachaches, headaches, fatigue, and all sorts of bodily complaints. With great trepidation, I decided to share my experience. I was fearful that my story, with its very bad ending, would sound morbid to them and would make things worse. Would I just convince them that they, too, were on their way to a tragic conclusion? I only had a few short seconds to decide what to do.

So slowly, and trying to hold back my own tears, I told them of our experiences. Details were not important, but substance was. I told them my son, who was in high school during most of the difficult years, had experienced similar health problems to those Anthony was now experiencing. I talked continuously for about fifteen minutes, which could have been a problem given the whole visit was only allotted fifteen minutes on my hectic patient schedule. Medicine today often doesn't give us the time we need with our patients—there's too much pressure to "move patients through." But on that day, with my patient struggling with symptoms I was all too familiar with, time really didn't matter at all. As I was speaking, Anthony affixed his eyes to mine and no longer was interested in the floor. His mother also listened intently, not only to see the effect of the story on her son, but likely thinking about herself as well.

Looking back now I can't remember the exact words I said, but in general I know I talked about loss, grieving, love, needing to carry on despite hardship. I talked about the "brain-gut connection" and how our minds and bodies are closely interconnected, and that thinking of them as separate entities often blinds us to the true triggers and causes of disease. There was a good explanation for Anthony feeling the way he was, and I believed it was unlikely he was suffering from any severe illness. We talked about strategies for coping with the physical and emotional demands, and the importance of caretakers taking care of themselves as well. That may be the hardest lesson of all for any of us, including me and my son, to accept. It is okay to give yourself a break. We talked about finding someone to talk to on a regular basis, the importance of exercise, being with friends, and getting away at times without feeling guilty. The mood in the room softened, the 900-pound gorilla released. We all breathed again.

I wondered how things would go that night when they got home. Their reality would be the same. But would they be a bit stronger, and perhaps more accepting of the situation? Would some of the resentfulness or anger or fear or guilt that had triggered Anthony's physical symptoms abate? Would they heed my advice about arranging for a therapist to help him sort through all of the emotions and turmoil compounding his adolescence—a period of life inherently filled with its own emotions and turmoil? This would test the resilience and inner fortitude of this young man as it did my own son in a very parallel situation.

I felt exhausted after their visit. I hoped that my patient's burden was lessened, if only for a short time. In telling him of my family's struggle with the mind-body connection, how the stress my son and I experienced had affected us physically, I reflected on how doctors must at all times be conscious of how very human we are, and how our own life stories can help, and be helped, by the life stories of our patients.

But it was still early in the day and I had many more patients on my schedule, which was now even further backed up. As cathartic for me as the flashbacks to my own life had been that morning, I needed to put them aside, tuck them away in a drawer, and move on. I hope someday Anthony will get to a place where he can do the same.

DATE OF EVENT: EARLY 2010s

The Miracles of Grace and Patience

Kathleen M. Gutierrez, MD

"**J**" is just a little boy. At the time this is written, he has been in the hospital, hundreds of miles from his home, for seventy-six days and counting. His father is here, too, every day, twenty-four hours a day. J was born with a condition causing the bones in his skull to fuse together too soon, resulting in an unusually shaped head. He also has *hydrocephalus*, an abnormal collection of fluid in his brain resulting from a blockage of the normal drainage pathways for brain fluid. To remove the excess fluid from his brain where the pressure could cause further damage, he requires a tube running under the skin all the way from his brain to his abdomen. As if all of that wasn't enough, he is hard of hearing and also requires a tube inserted directly through the skin of his neck into his *trachea* (windpipe) to help him breathe.

As a result of his medical conditions, he has had a dozen major surgeries, forty or more minor procedures, and many hospital admissions since birth. Now, he is back in the hospital with a severe fungus infection. We—J, his father, his surgical and medical teams—have worked together through this long winter-through-spring hospitalization to battle the tenacious germ. A few times we have been optimistic that finally the two strong drugs and multiple procedures to clean out the infection resulted in cure. But our hopeful hubris is always short-lived as new areas of swelling arise on his battered young face, and the search for the germs' elusive hiding place begins again. The bone and tissue in his forehead have poor blood supply, restricting our ability to get the medicines where they need to be. The drugs seem to have "stunned" the germ, which when removed from the affected areas no longer grows in the test tube, but we still see its face at random intervals when tissue is viewed under the microscope.

Almost every physician on our team has cared for J at some time over these many weeks. Our weekly clinical care conference, where our doctors meet to share ideas that might aid in our treatments, inevitably begins with questions about J. "How is he this week?" "Are there new ideas or words of wisdom?" "What can we do to best help them?"

J and his father have inserted themselves deeply into the hearts of all who care for them. Their faces drift into consciousness even when we are not at the hospital: on the drive home, in line at the grocery store, on a morning walk. We all read and re-read J's medical history searching to understand the anatomy of his exhausted body, to understand where this germ lurks unseen. We consult the sparse medical literature describing cases of refractory infections to guide us in constructing an effective treatment plan that keeps side effects to a minimum.

Despite the difficulty eradicating this cruel infection, J and his father are patient and courageous. Bad news—of which there has been plenty—is met with disappointment but remarkable equanimity. J attends "hospital school" every day, where he is a good student. He remains polite and respectful to all of his caregivers. He is such a brave little boy. He cries only in anticipation of the painful but necessary changes of his bandages. His beautiful smile, sense of humor, and kindness lighten our days and lift our ache. His father is a thoughtful advocate for his son's care and his calmness settles like a blessing on our shoulders. We ask them, how is it possible to suffer so, to live with setback after setback, but still convey such extraordinary light and love to each other and to all of us who meet you? Their answer of course is that for them there is no other choice except to respond with grace—and one can only imagine how difficult this must be.

At our weekly clinical conference, one of our fellows, a trainee, spoke of J. She reported another major procedure on the immediate horizon to remove bone pieces from J's forehead in the persistent battle to eradicate this infection. To conclude her presentation, our trainee said, "Their patience is a miracle." And so it is. For the surgical and medical teams working alongside J and his dad, struggling to accomplish what we want for them, their grace and courage are truly miraculous and inspiring.

Postscript: It is now over a year since this essay was originally written and, much to our great joy, J is doing well. Although we still follow him for any setbacks, he has had none. He has not required additional surgery or new therapy in all that time, and it is our great hope that the grace and patience he and his father have shown will finally herald a cure.

DATE OF EVENT: 1981

Unequal Twins

Edward J. Goldson, MD

*A*h, *little person, you are trying so hard!* Sean was one of fraternal twins born at about thirty-two weeks gestation, two months premature. Although he was a little bigger than his twin sister, he struggled more medically. At one point he required help breathing with a mechanical breathing machine, had an ongoing dependence for additional oxygen, did not feed well, and had trouble maintaining his temperature. In contrast, his twin sister was a superstar, breathing room air, feeding normally, and in an open crib growing just as expected.

Sean's parents and older sister were devoted to the twins, but Dad had a special relationship to Sean. Dad had always wanted a son and was very excited about the baby. He also knew that this would be his wife's last pregnancy as she had been very ill carrying these babies.

Time passed and Sean's twin sister was discharged home, now at the healthy weight expected for a full-term baby. She was healthy in every other way also. Sean, however, continued to have challenges with breathing, weight gain, and temperature control. It also became apparent to those of us caring for Sean that his father was also having difficulties with his son's slow progress. Dad began to visit Sean less frequently. This can mean many things in the context of a sickly baby, but those of us caring for Sean were concerned that his father was disengaging from the baby and wondered how he would accept the infant once he came home. Would Sean meet his father's hopes and expectations?

To our collective relief, Sean finally began making progress. He was able to maintain his temperature, began eating better and gaining weight, seemed more alert, and was able to wean from his supplemental oxygen. At discharge time we gathered the family together. As part of the discharge protocol, I performed a complete neonatal assessment and physical examination of Sean with his family attentively observing. It was a wonderful time, but a scary time for the parents. Would the assessment find Sean *truly* ready to go home? The excitement was palpable as Sean was able to accomplish all of the tasks presented to him and he looked and acted like a healthy baby. It was hard to believe, considering how difficult the days and weeks before had been.

At the end of the assessment Sean was wrapped snugly in a warm blanket and presented to his father, a happy day for all. Afterward, we saw him only once or twice in follow-up as the family lived far from the hospital. Several years passed and the family was in Denver for a visit and happened to be in the lobby of the hospital just as I was. We had a warm reunion filled with hugs and greetings. As the kids' mother wandered off in the lobby to corral the children, their father turned to me and asked if I remembered that "exam" I had performed the day of Sean's discharge. Of course I did!

Father turned to me and said, "I don't know if you realize it, but that day you give me my son." My sense was, until that examination demonstrating Sean's wonderful and hard-earned abilities, he feared he would be taking home a son who was not "normal"; a child who would not go fishing or play ball with his father or participate in all the father-son activities he looked forward to sharing with his son.

And then, as if on cue, Sean came running down the hall to his beaming dad, kicking a soccer ball, a perfectly normal miracle of a child. I was almost as proud as Sean's dad, proud at how we had all worked together to help establish this healthy, loving family.

It's often hard to know the exact ingredients that go into a dramatic medical turnaround like Sean's, but I was grateful to have been there to see it.

DATE OF EVENT: 2002

Maybe Justin Will
Be Different

Jeffrey S. Hyams, MD

I remember it was a Friday afternoon, ending a very long and difficult week. I was sleep-deprived, crabby, and just generally not in the mood to be cheerful. I am a gastroenterologist, a specialist in stomach and intestinal disorders, and when my beeper went off informing me of a consult in the pediatric intensive care unit (PICU) I knew it wasn't going to be good news. Just a name and age appeared, with no clinical details: Justin, three years old. I went up to the third floor, swiped my badge, and entered the eighteen-bed PICU that usually presented me with sensory overload. I opened the chart to read about a young boy, totally well until a few days ago, who had developed abdominal pain and vomiting. He had initially been felt by his family to have a viral illness, especially after receiving phone reassurance from his doctor. But when his condition worsened, the family took Justin to the local emergency room. Justin couldn't stop vomiting, the pain got more intense, and he became listless.

After a number of hours there, with his clinical condition deteriorating, he was transferred to our hospital where further testing suggested a bowel obstruction. He was brought to the operating room in the middle of the night and found to have a *volvulus,* with massive bowel damage caused by lack of blood flow to the bowel. A volvulus occurs when the intestine twists upon its nutrient blood supply and is deprived of oxygen. In young children, a congenital abnormality of the arrangement of intestinal loops, called *malrotation,* predisposes to volvulus. While some bowel loss is survivable, Justin had lost over 90 percent of his small intestine and was left with very little hope. He was unstable with low blood pressure, poor urine output, and fever. The immediate prognosis was guarded at best, and long-term it seemed unlikely he would ever be able to survive independent of intravenous (given into a vein) nutrition or without a bowel transplant.

After finishing my chart review I entered Justin's darkened room, illuminated only by the green glow of the monitor. His little body rhythmically moved slightly with each breath entering his lungs from the ventilator (breathing machine). All of his muscles were paralyzed so he wouldn't fight back against the breathing machine that was keeping sufficient oxygen flowing to his body. Multiple intravenous catheters (tubes in his veins) were giving him fluids, blood, antibiotics, and powerful medicines to sustain his blood pressure, which was dangerously low.

Huddled in the corner of the room were his parents, trying to understand why their normal toddler of several days ago was now desperately fighting for his life. My unenviable job was to tell them that even if he survived the present situation he was likely to require difficult, complicated, and expensive care for the rest of his life, and even then he had a good chance of dying. So I took a deep breath, introduced myself, and sat down beside them. I explained he had lost a large amount of his bowel, it was unlikely he would ever be able to sustain himself and grow normally eating food by mouth again, and he would be dependent upon intravenous nutrition. He would be prone to having serious infections with an intravenous catheter in his veins, and long-term intravenous nutrition (called *hyperalimenation fluid*) could cause his liver to fail. One day, if we were lucky, he would have a small bowel transplant and then would require anti-rejection medications the rest of his life. The five-year survival for small bowel transplantation at that time, 2002, was at best 50 percent. But, like I always did during these conversations, I never removed hope that maybe Justin would be different. I told them that even though I could not honestly be optimistic at that moment, surgery and medicine are powerful tools with which we'd try to make him better. I added that sometimes miracles happen and events turn out different than we expect.

When I returned to the hospital on Monday, I went to the ICU first and talked to the resident (physician-in-training) on call to hear about the weekend. She told me that Justin had done surprisingly well and was already being weaned off the ventilator. Over the next couple of weeks Justin had the usual setbacks of fevers, blood test abnormalities, and the like, but overall his progress was strong. As the acute surgical care was ending, the bulk of Justin's intestinal "rehabilitation" now fell into my lap as the pediatric gastroenterologist. I have always considered *short-gut syndrome*, the condition Justin now had after most of his intestine had been removed, to be the epitome of intellectual challenge of my field. I have referred to it as the "champagne" of pediatric gastroenterology. Expertise in nutrition, gastrointestinal and liver physiology, kidney function, infectious diseases, and psychology are all required to optimize the care of these children.

So we started the process slowly by giving very small amounts of a specialized formula, which has already been predigested, through a tube inserted in the stomach directly through the abdominal wall (called a *gastrostomy*). This technique, known as trickle feeds, exposes the minimal remaining intestine to key nutrients and stimulates the growth of new intestinal cells. Our only hope was that over the ensuing years a process called *intestinal adaptation* would allow the intestine to grow in length (he was only three years old so there was still time for growth) and, more importantly, the remaining surface of the intestine would increase its ability to absorb nutrients.

Justin went home and I saw him weekly for the next several months. Our progress was quicker than I expected, and by six months he was receiving about 40 percent of his daily calories through the gastrostomy tube and the rest intravenously. Being a normal toddler, he wanted to eat but we had to be very careful because even small amounts of regular food caused him to get severe diarrhea. He didn't have sufficient intestinal cells to digest and process regular food. At every visit Justin's family asked if he would ever get off the intravenous nutrition and my reply was I wasn't sure, but he was already doing better than I ever expected.

Justin grew, gained weight, and became an otherwise normal child. At age nine, defying any sane prediction of his eventual course, we were able to remove the intravenous catheter through which he had been receiving nutrition and sustain normal growth on the gastrostomy tube feedings into his stomach. We were even able to allow him small amounts of regular food by mouth. The removal of the intravenous catheter was a momentous event, a cause for celebration, as he now had the opportunity to go into the ocean with his family when they traveled to the beach each summer. To Justin, the ability to swim in the ocean was more important than this newfound intestinal freedom.

He did well for a number of years, but at age thirteen his growth rate started to slow and he was not keeping up with his peers. It appeared as if the amount of nutrition he could absorb was not enough to foster a growth spurt associated with puberty. After long negotiation we finally were able to convince Justin, his family, and ourselves that an intravenous catheter needed to be reinserted for extra calories. It was, and things went well for about two months before he developed a clot in the vein in which the catheter was placed and the catheter had to be removed. The clot was large enough that his face swelled and we had to give him powerful medicine to help dissolve the clot. But he got through it fine and we finally were able to adjust his feedings to get him to slowly gain weight again.

So now we are a dozen years following that eventful day when I first met Justin and his family. As a fifteen-year-old now, he has not only defied all of my initial predictions but thrown them far, far away. Justin has survived, and even thrived, a bright light at the end of what has been a very long tunnel for him and his family.

I have taken care of other children in similar circumstances, used the same passion and knowledge on their cases, and yet none have had this degree of medical success. Indeed, Justin did turn out different than what we expected.

I still don't know why he has been different than the rest. It wasn't anything I did differently or more brilliantly.

As I told the family those many years ago, sometimes miracles happen.

DATE OF EVENT: 1985

My First Patient

Robert J. Buys, MD

At last I had finished all my education. Four years of medical school, a year of internship, three years of residency in ophthalmology (the specialty providing medical and surgical care of the eyes), and two years of subspecialty fellowship training in diseases and surgery of the retina and vitreous had prepared me for that first real day of my professional career. Or so I thought.

I will never forget my first patient.

Kim was twenty-four and blind when we first met. She had given birth to a healthy baby boy a year before and never seen his face. The pregnancy had caused her diabetes to go on a rampage and resulted in a sudden loss of vision. Diabetes can have catastrophic and often permanent consequences to the eye. It does this by destruction of the blood supply to the retina, the lining in the back of the eye required for vision. As the blood vessels die away, the eye will try making new vessels to replace them. Unfortunately, these new blood vessels do not restore the lost blood supply and can break, causing bleeding into the jelly of the eye (called the *vitreous*).

Or worse, the blood vessels can scar and pull on the underlying retina, causing detachment, which was the case with Kim. One eye had this so-called *tractional retina detachment*, and such significant loss of blood supply I considered it hopeless. The other eye was not far behind; diabetic retinopathy is nothing if not democratic, affecting both eyes equally given enough time. In this race against time I was losing—badly.

I tried to operate on the worst of Kim's two eyes and the result was what I'd feared. Even though I was able to get anatomical success, reattaching the retina to the back of the eye, the retina had no blood supply and the eye quickly became painful and unable to see light. Reluctantly, I had no choice but to remove the eye.

That still left her with one eye, even though she could barely detect light. We had to go back to the OR and try to salvage it. My expectation was that with or without surgery the chance of success was grim. The night before the surgery she called me, hysterical—how could she go ahead with surgery when the other eye had done so badly? I rushed to the hospital and sat by her bedside. I held her hand and did my best to reassure her this time would be different. But who was I fooling? I knew her only chance for any vision at all was surgery, but in my heart I agreed with her—it was undoubtedly futile.

The morning of surgery arrived and we quietly went together to the OR. I held her hand again and whispered reassurances to her as the anesthesia took its effect. I took a moment before the surgery began to compose myself and prepare for the test ahead.

By end of the surgery I felt I had done as well as I could, but my assistant, who was also a retinal surgeon, was convinced we had lost the eye. I didn't know it then but he had gone out to Kim's parents in the waiting room and informed them of the expected bad result.

The memory of the next morning when I made rounds will be with me forever. I can still see her freckled face and strawberry blond hair, feel her sweet demeanor and the warmth of her personality all these years later. She was rubbing the edge of a coffee cup, turned to me and asked: "Does this mean I will be blind for the rest of my life?"

I could not bring myself to tell her what I feared. "I am not giving up, let's wait and see what happens." It was as honest a response as I could come up with.

The next few weeks were the hardest. She would come to the office disheveled, depressed. Her vision remained limited to barely seeing hand motions, but the front of the eye remained free of new blood vessels—a good sign—and the pressure inside her eye remained normal, also a good sign. She asked if it would be okay for her to call me at home if problems arose, and I quickly agreed. And she did call—whenever she was afraid, or just needed to cry and release her emotions. I did not want to be anywhere else but at the other end of the phone in those dark and difficult times. To my mind, being there for the hard times with your patients is what being a doctor is all about. When she hung up after those calls I cried, too.

Then one night everything began to change. I have played that call over in my mind a thousand times and it all comes rushing back as I write this.

"I am not sure, but I see something red and blurry. I think it is the numbers on my alarm clock."

Two days later she came to the office. I loved calling out her name myself in the waiting room and watching her little boy hop up and run to hug me. When I saw her that day she was completely different, all dressed up, makeup on. I should have known by the way she walked into the examination room that things had changed.

I checked her vision, first to light, then with the letter "E" on a piece of paper a foot away. She had never been able to see that in the entire time I had known her.

"That is the letter 'E', upside down. But the one down the hall (which was twenty feet away) is normal." She then ripped off the letters of the eye chart all the way down to 20/60 vision—not quite perfect, but a huge improvement!

I was stunned and my office staff was momentarily silent. Then a huge roar went up, followed by cheers and laughter. She smiled at me and I could not help the tears that rolled down my face. Nurses and techs hugged her.

When my turn for a hug came she said, "Who are you? You cannot be Dr. Buys." She had never seen me before; I guess I look different than I sound.

After that it was easy from the eye standpoint. She maintained her vision, even got a limited driver's license, and went back to work. Sometimes before an exam she would pop out her glass eye, rub it off, and put it back in. "That should help," she would say with a smile.

But tragically, her diabetes remained aggressive and picked her body parts off one at a time. First her legs, then her kidneys, then her heart. Just before the end I went to see her in the hospital. Several years had passed and she had gratefully and joyfully watched her son grow up, maintaining excellent vision even though every other organ in her body failed.

Kim's miraculous result sustained me through the years whenever I faced grim problems in other patients. When I reflect on my practice and my patients, she is always the first out of the box; my first patient continues to be my most poignant clinical memory. Even during the difficult times, when her diabetes ravaged her, that warm, happy, funny girl I met all those years ago was still there through it all, for her son and her family.

And for me, she remains forever so.

DATE OF EVENT: 1979

Thirty-Six

Michael D. Lockshin, MD

Thirty-six years ago, I did not yet understand how special Michelle was. At that time she was a child, just thirteen years old. I was young, too, in a professional sense, since I was a new attending (supervising) physician. Trained in adult *rheumatology* (the specialty caring for patients with arthritis, autoimmune disorders, and other diseases of the joints and muscles), I did consultations on children only because, at that time, our hospital did not yet have pediatric rheumatologists. I didn't like to consult on children. They tended to scream when I entered their rooms. Also, as a new father, I felt personal anguish when I saw an ill child.

But Michelle was different. She turned the doctor-patient role around, immediately putting me at ease, laughing as her arms and legs would suddenly and uncontrollably twist and jerk, thinking her illness funny. "My body is controlled by ghosts," she giggled. I, the dour consultant, laughed with her. She had a nervous system disorder called *chorea* that caused involuntary muscle movements. Her chorea, in turn, was caused by *systemic lupus erythematosus* ("lupus"), a debilitating autoimmune disease where a patient's immune system attacks her own body.

My consultation finished, I made a recommendation to her pediatrician. He disagreed with me, leading to a kind of debate that involved Michelle's parents. Our different opinions so discomfited the parents that they took Michelle to another rheumatologist elsewhere in town. It was an amicable transition, since he was a colleague and friend, and also because he agreed with my plan and not her pediatrician's. Michelle's parents, the new doctor, and I were all active in a lupus advocacy group, so we saw one another often, and thus I watched Michelle grow. Her doctor also gave me clinical updates from time to time.

Michelle did well with treatment. She had an easy adolescence, graduated from college, enjoyed a romance or two, traveled, and began a creative job with a drama group. She lived a life that was not dictated by her illness.

Unfortunately, a few years later her disease caught up with her with a vengeance. She developed inflammation in her kidneys, then had a heart attack at age twenty-eight, coronary bypass surgery, and a second heart attack five years after that. It was then that I first began to realize how special she really was.

This is what happened. After the second heart attack Michelle developed heart failure, from which she seemed to recover. She asked her other doctor if she was well enough to attend a family event for which she would have to travel from New York to the West Coast. He said yes. She went.

A few days later telephone calls came, four in rapid succession, each more urgent than the last. The first came from Michelle's father, the others from an intensive care specialist, a cardiologist, and a kidney specialist—I forget the exact sequence—all in that Western town. Michelle was in an intensive care unit (ICU) there, desperately ill. The doctors described the problem and asked me how I would treat her lupus. Her parents asked if I would transfer her to New York. They thought her other doctor had given dangerously bad advice and wanted me to assume her care.

I made the necessary arrangements, and then waited for our ICU to call to tell me that she had arrived.

✧ ✧ ✧

This is a Talmudic tale. God is so angry at the wickedness of men that he decides to destroy all mankind. But he reconsiders, deciding not do so for this reason: at any one time there exist thirty-six people on earth who are so righteous that he will not destroy them. To spare just these thirty-six righteous ones, God forgives all the others. According to the tale, the number is magical. There are always thirty-six such people on earth. They are called, in Hebrew, the *lamed vav* (thirty-six) *tzadikim* (holy ones). No one, not the *tzadikim* nor anyone else, knows who they are.

Or almost no one.

There are two possible ways by which one might recognize a holy one, a *tzadik*. The first is through intuition: you see someone do or say something so extraordinarily good that you intuit from the action—you can never know for certain—that the person is a *tzadik*. The second way is that you sense (by which of your five senses, or if by a sixth sense, I do not know) the brief flight of angels that escorts a *tzadik* to heaven when the *tzadik* dies.

There is one remaining part of the tale. The brief moment between a *tzadik*'s death and his or her arrival in heaven is the only time at which there are only thirty-five *tzadikim* on earth. The instant the deceased *tzadik* enters heaven, God appoints a new one, and once again there are thirty-six.

✧ ✧ ✧

Fifteen years have passed since the day that Michelle flew back to us and to our ICU. I am still a doctor, not so young now. In my long career, though I have met impressive and powerful people, only once did I think I might have met a *tzadik*. That was the evening Michelle came to our ICU.

I saw there a young woman, weakened by severe illness, exhausted after a transcontinental flight, nearly completely hidden by dialysis tubes and arterial lines and a breathing mask tightly affixed to her bloated face. Her eyes were drawn; she was much more ill than I had ever seen her before. Though her eyes were closed, she did not sleep. She opened her eyes and gazed hazily at me as I entered the room. Every doctor knows the look that I describe.

Motioning me close, she whispered, "Are my parents okay? They must be so frightened."

Near death, exhausted, broken by lifelong disease, yet the first thing she says is, "Are my parents okay?" Her main concern at this most dire moment in her life was the well-being of her parents? How can anyone so ill think that way? How beyond selfless is it possible to be?

Many things happened to Michelle over the next decade and a half. She had more dialysis; a kidney transplant; abnormal heart rhythms requiring an implanted defibrillator that restarted her heart from time to time when it stopped beating; episodes of bone marrow failure; recurrent heart failure; inflammation of her pancreas; fracture of the vertebrae in her neck requiring surgical fusion; a period of six hospitalizations in six months for medication adjustment. As if that was not enough, there were also conversations and consultations about her having yet another kidney transplant and then a heart transplant.

As she did at thirteen when I first met her, Michelle laughed at the indignities her bad health had caused, at the ghosts inside of her. When she felt well, she beamed as she talked to me about the play she and her boyfriend had produced. She looked and felt beautiful in her elegant gown as she passionately spoke at a lupus fundraiser each year. She appeared in educational videos on behalf of the S.L.E. Lupus Foundation/Lupus Research Institute and served on their committees. She was a tireless advocate for others with her devastating disease. She was excited to think of a future post-transplant day. After all she had been through, and after all these years, Michelle still made me laugh.

✧ ✧ ✧

There came then, of course, the last telephone call.

Michelle collapsed at home, her father said. The defibrillator in her heart fired but to no avail. The ambulance with its emergency medical technicians came but were unable to revive her. I had known Michelle for thirty-six years. Though I had laughed with her just a week or two before, I was terribly saddened but not surprised by the call.

Like most doctors do, I suppose, I thought about Michelle for all that night—and for many more nights and years afterward. I thought about the many times we had chatted, in my office or beside her hospital bed, about her worries for her parents, and sometimes about her worries for a problem of a friend. I thought about her altruism and her advocacy. How was it possible for anyone to be so selfless, let alone someone whose life was so filled with physical pain and challenges? Fifteen years ago, standing at Michelle's bedside in the ICU, I had an intuition that I could not put into words. The night her father called, I did not sense a flight of angels. The Talmudic tale may or may not be true—I have no way to verify. But I do believe that, for a very brief moment as I spoke to her father that dreadful night, there were only thirty-five *tzadikim* in the world.

12

Back to
the Beginning

All of the physicians contributing the poignant and inspirational essays in this book began their careers as medical students: unsure, insecure, and frightened. The transition from student to professional in any career requires a significant effort on the part of the trainee as well as by those doing the training. But because of the high stakes involved in medical careers, with patients' lives and families' strength and stability on the line, a successful transition is all the more important.

This final essay, written by one of our nation's leading medical educators, describes the miraculous transformation to professionalism that all physicians must undergo if they are to be privileged to experience, and contribute to, the types of miracles described in all of the other essays in this book.

DATE OF EVENT: 1980–2015

A Doctor's Work:
The Miracle of Professional
Transformation

Carol L. Storey-Johnson, MD

I am a medical educator, dedicating my career to the training and growth of future physicians. In that context, it is my responsibility and privilege to help turn trainees into physicians, in every sense of that word. Effecting such a transformation is vital for the future of health care. Without it, physicians will be no different than technicians, computers, or robots, and perhaps less compassionate than any of those.

The diversity of students now entering medical school is truly a wonderful thing to behold. Nearly half of the members of entering medical school classes are women, and, while the task is not easy, progress is also being made in ethnic and cultural diversity. I have often pondered the assumptions we make about these young future physicians as they enter our august halls of learning and begin their path to becoming successful and outstanding physicians and scientists. There is so much for them to learn and, it seems, so little time to learn it all. They not only have to acquire an extensive fund of knowledge to successfully treat patients, but they must also learn how to act and comport themselves as physicians. My observation has been that this behavioral transformation into the professional role is often as, or even more, challenging for them as learning the science of medicine. I have always been intrigued by how our students learn this. How do they transform their personal selves to become professionals, and how can we help them with that task?

Times have changed. I recall that, during my own medical training, I was expected to take full responsibility for my actions, learning, and professional growth. The specific route to "turning into a doctor" was not taught in classroom sessions at that time. For the most part we learned by observing older role models (senior doctors) and trainees close to us in years who supervised our day-to-day activities. I remember that "pulling yourself up by your bootstraps" was clearly the work ethic of the day. Help would be available if I asked, but it was more generously offered if I demonstrated I could almost do it all myself. I was expected to go out and learn the various disciplines in medicine, with that phrase that educators now find frightful, "See one, do one, teach one" always in the back of my mind. You had to learn new things as soon as possible—and be fully ready for the next event. Requirements for further training and career advancement and recognition were that you did the right thing, as best you could, and you didn't hide anything. If all that went well, you were promoted to the next training level. Somehow, it seemed a given that your personal and professional integrity were always up front, on the line, and requiring more and more polish and effort over time. And you gave of yourself and your time unselfishly in your pursuit of the highest quality of patient care. So much of what was expected of us for professional growth in those days was passively conveyed.

Today, the transformation to a professional physician is more directly and explicitly addressed in the curriculum, usually in the form of "doctoring courses." When I teach new students about their professional growth, I often refer to the writings of Frederic Hafferty, PhD, among others, who wrote about the ways in which we learn to comport ourselves as physicians within our learning environments. In one eloquent and oft-quoted article, Hafferty wrote about three curricula learners face every day: the explicit curriculum (the goals and information we teach the learners in our classrooms); the implicit curriculum (an informal and highly interpersonal curriculum of "dos and don'ts" that learners encounter on the floors of our teaching hospitals and medical college corridors); and the hidden curriculum (those messages that institutions send almost subliminally when we examine, for example, what the institutions value, who they reward, and how their policies are written).

Hafferty also noted that these three curricula are not always aligned. Disturbingly, the implicit and hidden curricula are extremely powerful and can overshadow the explicit teaching we do. For example, what we teach in our classrooms is not what students may see in our teaching arenas—students may witness disrespect among colleagues, or lack of alacrity when caring for certain patient populations. These arise more frequently than we would like to admit if we were being truthful, as evidenced by the accounts our trainees report routinely to their teachers during debriefings of their clinical and teaching experiences. It is what we see of the actions of others who are more senior than us (and evaluating us!), and our immediate day-to-day role models, that has great impact on how we behave in similar situations, and as future physicians.

As I look back on my own career, I consider myself to be a fortunate beneficiary of these three curricula. I had excellent role models; doctors whose behaviors I could emulate without a second thought, those who were re-spected by all and held in highest regard. In general, the three curricula I encountered were aligned and pretty much in sync. But what if I had not been so fortunate? What if I encountered physicians and scientists willing to take shortcuts or misrepresent information? What if I personally came from a social and cultural environment where there was considerable variation in the levels of personal integrity that were expected? What if shortcuts were nearly always "okay" and the norm was just "Give me what I need" to perform or get to the next step? The competition and practices regularly faced in the business world are examples that come to mind—a haunting and disturbing thought as many physician practices have, of financial necessity, become businesses first, places of healing second.

When exams came around during my own days in training, I always equated my performance on a test with the development of an excellent knowledge base, one that would serve my patients exceptionally well. I was less assured of how to do things outside the classroom as I started internship training, but gradually this got better, easier, and I had excellent role models to see in action. I put forth my very best effort because I was certain that it would make me a better doctor. I had great faith that learning in depth, reading in depth, and being in command of as many potential ramifications of medical decisions as possible would prepare me well.

But in recent years, I realized that more and more students do not look at this as I did. I've often wondered what would have become of me as a physician if I had not had my underlying personal driving force or ambition to be deeply informed. After all, in this digital age, there are so many ways to come by information. Why should I have to read the entire chapter of the text? Wouldn't the synopsis be sufficient and get me to the answer more quickly? What if I had no role models in my family of individuals who purposely chose the longer, more challenging route to understanding material in depth? What would my professional transformation have been like then?

It was not until I became responsible for attesting to the professional maturation of medical students that I was able to see this issue in much sharper focus and with larger scope. The fact of the matter is that the value systems of our entering medical students seem, in many ways, more diverse than ever before, possibly reflecting their cultural diversity. These differences in values are revealed in one-on-one conversations with students when they come to our attention for "misdeeds," and also in seminars where, in a supportive environment, they are free to express a wide range of reactions they would have to specific circumstances. These differences do not lie with specific groups of students—gender, ethnicity, and age don't seem to matter. While I can't be certain, I suspect that prior life experience is what matters most.

The interactions I have had with medical students have provided me with deep insight and poignancy, and have guided my determination to help our trainees with their professional transformation when they need it or want it. And I share this as examples of the ways *miracles* in training can actually happen, if only we spend the time and invest in our trainees.

All of the students who are referred to me because of unprofessional or inappropriate behavior and interactions with others had performed admirably in the objective aspects of our clinical doctoring courses, in the examinations on history taking and physical examination, and on essays related to doctor-patient interactions and medical ethics. They knew what to say when asked directly. But they were having trouble with the "softer" part of professional transformation: they might have had disrespectful arguments with classmates, not shown up on time for rounds or conferences, or expressed dismissive attitudes to course preparation. They should not be doing these things, right? So, why were they? Some were distressed in their personal lives, and often we can find this out and help them. Others may have simply come from environments where these behaviors are accepted or tolerated, where the kinds of role models I was fortunate enough to encounter simply don't exist, and the students see their actions as innately acceptable and available for them to choose as they wish. Why should they change the way they are acting?

My interventions with these students are based on my observations over forty years in an academic medical center. When I meet with them to discuss these kinds of troubling issues, I encourage the student to be honest and truthful about the incidents they have been involved in, and I encourage them to capture the emotion of the moment and describe it as best as they can. And then I ask them if they are wondering why I, or others, are concerned about their behaviors. Interestingly, students are often surprised their behaviors have been noticed by the faculty and deans, and, even more disquieting, they often don't understand why we are concerned! So I offer to explain to them, simply and concisely, my philosophy of being a physician who behaves professionally.

To start, I explain that my intent is to help them to take advantage of all the wonderful future "perks" that go along with becoming a physician. One of the ways to maximize their advantages in the future is to be very aware of how their behaviors are affecting others. The cultivation of desirable behaviors, leaving behind those that are "off-putting," during the training process allows those behaviors to become professional habits they will carry forward with them into any arena they enter in the future. Whether patient care, laboratory or clinical research, or the vast array of alternative careers physicians can find themselves in today, professionalism is the key element for success and fulfillment. I tell them cultivating desirable behaviors allows all others (patients, colleagues, staff, visitors, etc.) in your environment to potentially accord you a special status, respect, and acceptance that can ease your way forward in your career. Your opinion will be sought, you will be on the short list considered for new opportunities for leadership, and many more doors will "magically" open up for you. Those who do not pay attention to the ways they affect others often lose out on opportunities for which another's selection, nomination, or recommendation of them is an important part of the process of advancement. I tell them if they don't become sensitive to the impact they have on others, they will someday wonder why they are not chosen for positions they seek. And they will feel less satisfied with their careers. The importance of making these desirable interpersonal behaviors habits of performance cannot be overemphasized, as they often transfer into the kinds of appropriate interpersonal behaviors young physicians will demonstrate in their patient interactions. Ultimately, the doctor's relationship with his or her patients is the true metric by which a physician's merit and standing should rest.

Remarkably, while the total number of these professionalism counseling conversations with students is relatively small, in more than half, the real miracle occurs soon thereafter. Within a week of graduation, or some other time during their final year of study, a small note appears under my office door. It typically says such things as: "Thank you, for the conversation we had, for the insights you provided . . . my world has improved greatly since our conversation . . . people now consider me for new opportunities and leadership . . . my patients seem pleased with my performance as their 'doctor' . . . I'm not sure this would have happened if we hadn't spoken about the importance of managing how other people see me . . . I had no idea how important this might be."

I have always been struck by the personal poignancy of these notes, and gratified that something as simple as straightforward and heartfelt conversations can have on a physician's future.

And so, in addition to the glorious experience of taking care of patients with myriad medical issues over my career, I have been even more blessed to have had the opportunity to provide guidance to medical students and physicians-in-training for over three and a half decades. When a professionally transformative event occurs for one of my students, I am ever grateful and cognizant of the large number of individuals who will benefit in the future from that single transformation. I am grateful that, along the way, I have been part of a more explicit curriculum that helps our students and physicians-in-training become the kind of professionals we would all select to take care of our family members.

Just as it is with caring for patients, we are also blessed in this work to care for those who come after us as physicians, as the Hippocratic Oath demands, and ensure their best health and well-being in preparation for their professional future.

For Hafferty's paper on the curricula for educating medical students, see:

Hafferty FW, "Beyond Curriculum Reform, Confronting Medicine's Hidden Curriculum," *Academic Medicine* 1998; 73: 403–407.

EPILOGUE

The editor of this book (Dr. Rotbart), as well as his literary agent (Lisa Leshne, the Leshne Agency) and contracts manager (Deirdre Smerillo, Smerillo Associates) are taking no income from this project. Rather, 100 percent of net proceeds from advances and royalties resulting from the sales of this book will be divided among charities designated by each of the contributing essayists and, in some cases, by their patients. Those charities are listed below in hopes readers might also consider supporting these worthy causes.

Alliance for Children

Alyn Children's Hospital

American Cancer Society

American Heart Association

American Lung Association of the Northeast

Arapahoe Philharmonic Orchestra

Arkansas Children's Hospital Foundation

Autism Speaks

Bay Area Cancer Connections

Big Brothers, Big Sisters

Catholic Relief Services

Children's Hospital Colorado Center for Cancer and Blood Disorders

Children's Hospital Colorado Child Health Clinic

Children's Hospital Colorado Foundation

Children's Hospital Colorado Special Care Clinic

Children's Hospital of Philadelphia Alumni Organization

Children's Hospital of Philadelphia Hematology Research

Christ Episcopal Church, Charlottesville, VA

Colorado I Have a Dream Foundation

Colorado Humane Society

CURE Childhood Cancer

DAT Minyan

Denver Dumb Friends League

Department of Pediatrics, Mount Sinai Medical Center, New York

Donate Life Northwest

Fast for Feast

Footwork, the International Podoconiosis Initiative

Joni and Friends

Head and Neck Cancer Strategic Initiative Fund, Ohio State University

The Health Wagon

Janet Weis Children's Hospital Pediatric Rural Trauma Initiative

Jersey Shore University Medical Center Foundation

Jewish Federation of Philadelphia

Juvenile Diabetes Research Foundation

Kawasaki Disease Foundation

Kempe Center for the Prevention of Child Abuse and Neglect

The Kempe Foundation

Lazarus Family Fund at the AMA Foundation

LDS Philanthropies

Living Room Ministries International, Kimbilio Hospice

Lucille Packard Children's Hospital

Lucille Packard Children's Hospital OB Family Fund

March of Dimes Foundation

Medical College of Wisconsin, CNS Infections Fund

National Brain Tumor Society

National Medical Fellowships

National Multiple Sclerosis Society

Natural Areas Conservancy, New York, NY

Operation Breakthrough

Reach Out and Read Colorado

Roundup River Ranch: A SeriousFun Children's Network Camp

Saint Rock Haiti Foundation

Samfund, Boston

Save a Child's Heart Foundation

Save the Children

Sensory Processing Disorder Foundation

S.L.E. Lupus Foundation/Lupus Research Institute

Society for Vascular Surgery Foundation

Special Fund of Rabbi Joshua Skoff at Park Synagogue, Pepper Pike, OH

Special Fund of Rabbi Wesley Gardenswartz at Temple Emanuel, Newton, MA

Surgical Infection Society Foundation for Education and Research

Tygerberg Children's Hospital Trust

University at Buffalo, School of Management

University at Buffalo, Jacobs School of Medicine and Biomedical Sciences

Washington University School of Medicine Dr. Frank O. Richards Medical Student Scholarship Prize

Wounded Warrior Project

ABOUT THE AUTHOR

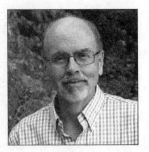

DR. HARLEY ROTBART has been a nationally renowned pediatric specialist, parenting expert, speaker, and educator for over three decades. He is Professor and Vice Chair Emeritus of Pediatrics at the University of Colorado School of Medicine and Children's Hospital Colorado. He is the author of more than 175 medical and scientific publications, and four previous books for general audiences: *940 Saturdays; No Regrets Parenting; Germ Proof Your Kids;* and *The On Deck Circle of Life,* which was endorsed by baseball Hall of Famer Cal Ripken Jr.

Dr. Rotbart has been named to *Best Doctors in America* every year since 1996, as well as receiving numerous other national and local awards for research, teaching, and clinical work. He serves on the Advisory Boards of *Parents Magazine* and *Parents.com* and makes numerous media appearances every year, including two recent satellite media tours with *American Idol* finalists to promote influenza prevention. Dr. Rotbart is a regular contributor to *Parents Magazine* and the *New York Times,* is a consultant to national and local media outlets, and writes his own blog at *www.harleyrotbart.com.* "Coach Harley" coached youth baseball and basketball for sixteen years, including eight years at the high school level.

Dr. Rotbart and his wife, Sara, live in Denver, Colorado, and are the parents of three grown kids, each a miracle in his or her own way.